Pressing RESET

Original Strength Forever

TIM ANDERSON

Pressing RESET™ - Original Strength Forever by Tim Anderson

Copyright © 2018, 2025 by Original Strength Systems, LLC.
All rights reserved.

Front cover design and interior photography
by Danielle "Dani" Almeyda

Published by OS Press Fuquay Varina, NC
Special thanks to Jetlaunch for all their help.

Paperback
ISBN- 978-1-963675-13-9
eBook
ISBN- 978-1-963675-14-6

Library of Congress Number available upon request.

CONTENTS

THIS IS MY STORY

I've always wanted to be Superman. I thought if I trained with weights, that would turn me into Superman. Weight training did make me stronger, and it gave me more confidence, but it also became an addiction, an identity really. I couldn't stop doing it even when it was causing me pain.

I had to do it. It was who I was—Timmy, the guy who always works out and never misses a day at the gym. It was a badge of honor. But it didn't make me Superman. In fact, after a few decades, it was wearing me down. My body was not feeling too great, and I started getting overuse injuries that I just couldn't get over.

The real reason I couldn't heal from those injuries is because I wouldn't let my body heal. I had to train. It was who I was. It's stupid, I know. But it was me.

One night, I felt pretty fragile and not at all like Superman. In desperation, I asked God to show me how to train to become bulletproof like Superman. And He did. He showed me how awesomely and wonderfully He designed the human being. He taught me how to move again and how to be truly strong from the inside out. His design is amazing.

I know that I know that I know we are made to heal. We are made to be strong and we are made to feel good. Our design to move and grow is evidence of this.

It's been over 14 years since I learned how to crawl again. Since then, I've been blessed to share our design all over the world. Seeing the spark of hope that ignites in someone's eyes never gets old when they discover they don't have to hurt, or when they experience the return of a movement they thought they had lost. It always makes me smile with gratitude.

If you don't know, you're not broken and don't have to be. Your body has a movement template tucked away inside it, designed to help you heal and live your best life. All you have to do is engage with it and move through it. This book will tell you how.

This is the fourth iteration of this book, not because the information has changed but because the wonder keeps revealing itself. I challenge you to read this and not discover the wonder of your body and its design. The information in this book is life-changing. But it won't just change your life; it will change the lives of those around you. When you live in your design, you live out the best version of yourself and make everything around you better.

If you don't believe me, just try Pressing RESET.

A SOBERING TRUTH

Movement and Exercise have risks associated with them. Research shows they can lead to being stronger, healthier, and happier. However, they can also lead to injuries or even death. It happens.

You should also know that doing nothing also has risks associated with it. Research shows that being sedentary can lead to sickness, weakness, frailty, depression, and anxiety. It can also make you more injury-prone and hasten your destination towards death. It happens.

Before beginning any exercise program, consult your trusted family physician. You should also consult your trusted family physician before engaging in any sedentary lifestyle.

"Every man dies, but not every man really lives."
—William Wallace, Braveheart

FOREWORD

As someone who has incorporated Original Strength (OS)'s Pressing RESET concepts into my practice as well as my own personal fitness, I have experienced its benefits first hand and witnessed it change the health and wellness of others. A few years ago, after a 16-mile trail run, I twisted my knee on dry creek bed. Afterward, I developed a recalcitrant knee pain that was confirmed on MRI as a chondral defect, a condition where permanent damage had been done to the cartilage in my knee.

As I have always done with my patients, I took a very biomechanical approach to my problem performing many of the best evidence-based exercises, modifying activity, and nutritional supplementation. My strength improved, but joint mobility with deep knee flexion, dead lifts, and kettle bell swings along with pain during running were still problematic. Mark Shropshire, a trusted strength and conditioning coach, introduced me to Tim's early works, *Becoming Bulletproof* and *Original Strength,* and I began working on "The Big Five" over the course of the following year. Since that time, I have returned to recreational running, completing a marathon and have helped many others return to activities that they didn't believe were possible.

After having success with Pressing RESET for my personal rehabilitation, my daughter incorporated Pressing RESET into a strength and conditioning program as an athlete with the USA Luge Team. It is often said that luge races are won in the summer, not in the winter. The preparation that gives an athlete a fast, powerful start, strong neck muscles needed to maintain optimal aerodynamics, and core control to steer a sled down an icy track at 90 mph, is a learned practice during the off season.[1] It is the commitment to the fundamentals of rocking, rolling, crawling, head control, and breathing that the good athletes become great athletes and when the Olympic hopeful becomes the Olympian.

Often times, something that starts as a personal interest has a way of influencing our professional interest. In 2013, the American Physical Therapy Association's Vision Statement for the Physical Therapy Profession defined movement as "a key to optimal living and quality of life for all people that extends beyond health to every person's ability to participate in and contribute to society."[2] Working with recreational and professional athletes, corporate and medical executives, and people with differing abilities, those who perform well are those who are able to master the transition from one movement pattern to another, achieving a desired functional outcome. Tim Anderson has taken the fundamental principles of movement system development strategies we innately employ as infants and toddlers and has reintroduced them to us as adults in a systematic manner.

Motor learning or skills acquisition can be broken down into two main categories: sequence learning and sensorimotor adaptation.[3] Often times, when learning new motor patterns, we will break the complex sequence into its constituent components and gradually integrate each component into its sequence. Take for instance, crawling. It is a complex movement that incorporates stability, mobility, and strength of the upper and lower limbs, scapulothoracic complex, and the lumbopelvic complex. Yet those complex movements are predicated by our horizontal gaze, head position, and breathing. Our sensorimotor adaptations such as the absence or presence of visual inputs, applied resistance or unweighting, or contact pressures all influence our response to altered limb dynamics that are associated with crawling.

With the use of a hierarchical approach to standard movement patterns of diaphragmatic breathing, head control, rocking, rolling, and crawling, Tim has provided a simple methodology for the therapist or exercise specialist to progress or regress a movement sequence to optimize motor learning. As a physical therapist that treats primarily orthopedic conditions and sports-related injuries, I have come to appreciate the essential role that proper movement system development has on my clients' ability to optimize their quality *IN* life.

I am grateful that Tim has been inspired to develop and refine the concepts of Original Strength. I admire Tim's passion for helping others and trust you will enjoy reading his latest inspiration: *Pressing RESET, Original Strength Forever.*

– Ken Johnson
PT Manager, Outpatient Rehabilitation Therapy Services
Administrator, Johns Hopkins Hospital/George Washington
University Orthopaedic Physical Therapy Residency
Johns Hopkins Hospital
Baltimore, Maryland

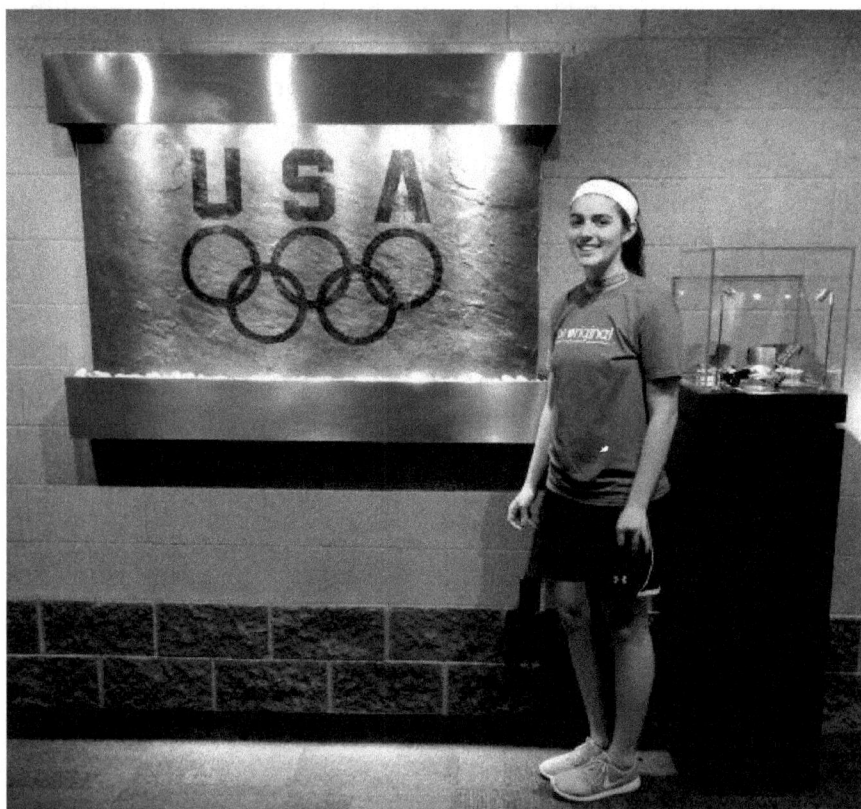

Camille Johnson, sporting OS shirt, at US Olympic Training Center
in Lake Placid, NY 2/25/2015

THE BEAUTY IN THE SIMPLICITY

– *Chip Morton,*
Strength and Conditioning Coach, Cincinnati Bengals

In my 30 years as a professional in the strength & conditioning field, I have witnessed, studied, and even used many of the ideas, techniques, and trends that characterize the ebbs and flows of our industry. Strength, stamina, power, flexibility/mobility, and the desire to maintain an appropriate body fat percentage, have been, and likely always will be, important training goals for many people.

Once during my first couple of years on the job as a strength coach in professional football, an older, more experienced coach told me that the most important aspect of a player's development to address in training was "movement". At the time, I dismissed it in favor of the more obvious responsibilities most often associated with my position, namely, strength and conditioning. Over the years, as I have matured and gained in wisdom and knowledge, my views have changed. I now understand and more fully appreciate the insight that older coach imparted to me years ago. We are in fact, "made to move."

Over the past few years, I have noticed a lot of attention and information has been devoted to helping people move *better*. We are told which mobility drills & stretches are best to perform and why, as well as how to perform them correctly; we're shown progressions, regressions, "flows", and the like. Within the variety of movement templates available on the Internet and in the literature, many are interesting to watch or read about. You can usually glean a few bits of usable information and even uncover common threads, or "truths", that weave their way through different programs. Some of the recommendations can be therapeutic, others may make you feel good, and even be fun to do. At some point, however, it seems to me, the more information we are presented with, the more complex things become, and the more difficult it is to discern what is best and how to put it all into practice on a consistent basis.

Moving well and what is required to attain that can be viewed from so many perspectives. There are many gifted individuals out there, demonstrating abilities forged from years of regular practice, perhaps with favorable leverages and the body dimensions necessary to master a particular skill set. As beautiful or enticing as they may appear, some movement prescriptions may not be a good fit for some people. This may stem from the amount of time and repetition required to achieve competency, or an inability to fit all the "moving parts" into an everyday schedule.

Finally, the prescription itself may simply not provide an appropriate entry point for certain individuals along their journey to reach their goals. The concept of "better movement" itself, is a quality unique to the individual to an extent, and lies along a continuum ranging from accessing the ranges of motion to improve day to day life, all the way to the ability to perform the movements required for elite athletic performance. Each one of us will define this quality differently, depending upon our individual needs and what we desire to accomplish.

The good news is God had already knit a movement "template" into each one of us. In fact, we progressed through parts or all of this progression as we developed and learned to move as infants. Re-introducing ourselves to our original movement plan is the foundation of Original Strength and it is the reason for its effectiveness. We are all "fearfully and wonderfully made" (Psalm 139:14) and some of the keys to unlocking better movement and health are already within us. They are there, in all of us, waiting to be re-discovered, and used to enhance our ability to live our lives to the fullest.

I was first introduced to Tim Anderson through Mr. John Brookfield, and shortly thereafter purchased a copy of his early work, **Becoming Bulletproof.** The material was easy to understand and use. Within the pages of that first book, I learned of the "RESETS" I could use to re-store my movement capability. These RESETS, namely diaphragmatic breathing, neck nods, rolling, rocking, crawling and cross-crawling, seemed logical and were simple to put into practice. No steep learning curve, no complex combinations that required great skill or coordination.

I will admit when I first tried some of the RESETS, I smiled and giggled a bit, "Baby-Crawling? Are you kidding me?" The giggles became "A-ha" moments more often as I regularly incorporated the RESETS into my daily schedule, in the mornings and before training. I noticed over the course of time, the range of motion I could attain when performing the RESETS improved and the movements themselves became more fluid and more intuitive. More importantly for me though, was the improvement in my "quality of life" activities, which at this point for me include playing alongside our children in whatever they are playing, meeting the physical requirements of my job, and lifting kettlebells.

Based on my personal experience with Pressing RESET, I believed incorporating it into our program would benefit our players' performance and ultimately, their well-being. So a couple of years ago, we invited Tim to visit our facility in order to introduce the fundamentals of Pressing RESET to my staff and me. My time with Tim added clarity to the concepts I had only read about up to that point, and refined my understanding of the RESETS as well as adding some variations we could use for our population, according to our specific needs. When he visited, Tim gave me a copy of the first edition of this book. Reading the information in *Original Strength* provided even greater insight, expanded my understanding of Pressing RESET, and opened the door to a deeper exploration of our intended ability to move and play!

As of this writing, I continue to learn more about the anatomical and physiological principles that gird up the Pressing RESET method, and as I do, I see the beauty in the simplicity of Original Strength's RESETS and the significant impact they can have on our amazingly intricate design. Over the past two years, we have incorporated the Pressing RESET method into programming for our players. Their initial reaction was similar to mine...giggles, but along with me, we Press RESET before most training opportunities and continue to explore and enjoy their impact on movement together.

In July of 2015, my family and I visited Tim and the OS Family in North Carolina to spend some quality time together and also for Tim to teach our children the fundamentals of Pressing RESET. Everyone from young children to professional athletes can perform the RESETS and benefit from them; I have witnessed it first-hand with people in my life who are important to me. Please allow me to encourage you to read *Pressing RESET, Original Strength Forever* and consider making the RESETS the basis of your movement practice. Re-build your movement and live the amazing life intended for you!

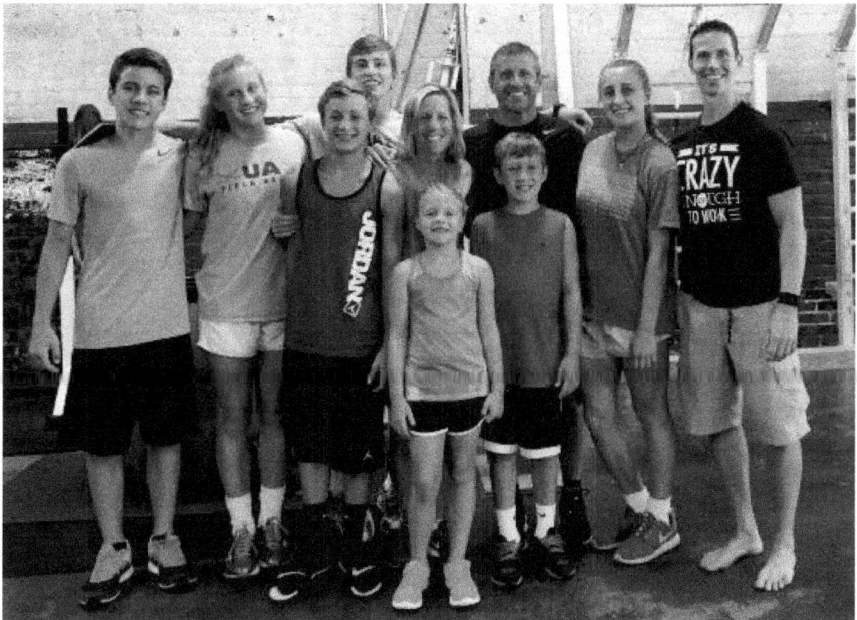

Tim Anderson & the Morton Family, July 2015

YOU ARE AWESOMELY AND WONDERFULLY MADE

You are the pinnacle of creation. No creature on earth rivals the wonder of a human being. Our bodies, minds, and souls make us wholly unique and completely wonderful. We are a creation with no limits other than the ones we place on ourselves.

From the very beginning of your existence, you were a blank slate of endless possibilities and potential. You were perfectly designed to possess all the enviable qualities of life: health, strength, creativity, courage, integrity, kindness, humor, intelligence, and compassion. You were to build these qualities through learning how to move. In fact, you were born with a movement template "preprogrammed" in your nervous system.

This program consisted of a series of reflexes and movements called the developmental sequence. As you grew through this sequence and mastered these movements you built your own brain, developed your mind, strengthened your body, and revealed your personality. The more you moved, the more you integrated your whole being. Your movements literally helped develop your entire being through integration - body, mind, and soul. They made you extremely strong and resilient from the center out, not just physically, but mentally and emotionally as well.

As a child, you experienced life through your design. Learning how to move through your developmental sequence you gained more strength, mobility, and stability every single day and each day you improved your ability to express yourself. By the time you were four years old, you were amazingly strong, creative, and resilient. You could run, laugh, play, climb, imagine, tumble, skip, wrestle, explore, and discover treasures every day. You were on a trajectory of robust health and wellbeing. But then life happened and your path to wholeness was altered.

Whether through an institutionalized education system, absorbing the fears of those around you, or being distracted and sedated with technology you learned how to *not move*. The very thing you were designed to do became the one thing the world discouraged. You learned how to be sedentary. From that moment, you began pruning away your foundation of expression potential.

If you're reading this book, you're probably an adult who feels "average" or less-than-average in your body. But you likely remember a time when you felt amazing; when you could run all day, laugh all night, and conquer whatever adventures the world invited you on. That amazing feeling *you* is the you that you were designed to be. It's also the *you* that you can still be. Though the modern world has tried to remove you from living in your design, it cannot remove your design from existing in you. And you cannot lose what you were born with - your original movement template. This means you can always build what you were created to have: strength, health, happiness, and wholeness.

Intuitively, you probably know this is true. If not, just think about it for a second. Humans are capable of living up to around 120 years. If that number defies your imagination or your conditioned logic meter, let's say that humans can easily live to the ripe old age of 80. Does it make any sense that the best, most robust days of our lives would be relegated from the age of 0 to 25? Is it possible that we are designed to grow weak and frail for the last 55 years of our lives? Shouldn't we at least be able to make it to 40 before everything starts to fall apart? But, if we could live to 120, and we can live to 80, wouldn't it make sense that we would be designed in such a way that we should be able to navigate through life with abundant strength at every age and through every season of life? Well, believe it or not, that is our design. The only reason we should lose our strength is because we have stopped living in our strength.

Your age should be a testimony of your resilience, not your frailty. Age should never be a "doom countdown." At worst it should only be an indicator of how many trips you were blessed to circle around the sun. In fact, if you didn't know how many circles you've made around the sun, it shouldn't matter. You're designed to feel and be strong and vibrant throughout all your sun cycles. Eagles soar until the day they die. We were meant to do the same thing.

Becoming weak and frail is what happens to us when we spend our lives being static, when we allow stress and fears to consume us. Becoming fragile is a result of not using our bodies in the ways they were designed to be used. Yes, many of us experience a life of aches, pains, lethargy, apathy, obesity, unsteadiness, high blood pressure, diabetes, and heart disease, but that does not mean we are supposed to. *You were not meant for any of these things!* Almost all of life's "issues" and "itis-es" could, or can, be combated, defeated, and even prevented, if we would revisit and engage in our original, pre-programmed movement patterns on a regular basis.

We were always intended to move, play and to engage in life. We were designed to enjoy life in health and strength. And we can. All we have to do is Press RESET and let our bodies heal.

You are indeed awesomely and wonderfully made.

How Do You Press Reset on Your Body?

You simply do what you did when you were a child: live in and through your design to move. The same movement template which was placed in you before you were born is still inside of you right now. This original movement program is waiting to carry out its original orders; to strengthen you from the inside out. This movement program never stops working. All you have to do is tap into it and use it.

By simply spending time on the floor and moving like a child, you are essentially Pressing RESET on your body and reestablishing your foundation of health and strength. Remembering how to breathe, controlling your head movements, rolling around on the floor, rocking back and forth, and even crawling around can re-establish wonderful reflexive connections throughout your entire body allowing you to express the strength, mobility, and vitality that has always been yours to have and express.

I know this sounds crazy, but it is crazy enough to work! By the end of this book you will know what I'm saying is true.

If you want to have a resilient body, one that will serve you well for a lifetime, start moving like you did when you were a child. It is amazing what a difference this will make in your body and soul. Engaging in and relearning your "child-like" movements is the key to turning back the hands of time and reclaiming the body you were meant to have.

Before you dismiss this as "too good to be true," consider that your body is designed to heal itself from sickness, disease, and injury. Being weak and fragile is essentially an injury to both your soul and your body. Reversing the weakness and frailty of age, neglect, and false beliefs is simply the body's way of healing itself. That is what happens when we Press RESET.

Intuitively, you know that life is meant to be enjoyed. You also know that if you really want to enjoy your life, you need a healthy body. Being sick, injured, and in pain should not be the norm or the status quo. And it certainly should not be a result of time simply passing us by! This may be hard to imagine right now, but even in our 90s, we should be able to sprint without having knee pain. We should be able to pick up a suitcase without hurting our backs. We should be able to grab something out of the back seat of our car without tearing a rotator cuff. We should be resilient, always, at any age.

"I try to get up and be productive, and don't let the old man in."
—Clint Eastwood

You are not supposed to be weak or fragile. Refuse to accept these conditions. Move and heal. No matter your body's current state, you can start where you are, begin Pressing RESET, and regain your original strength. Everything you need to become resilient and strong is already inside you, waiting to be tapped into again.

You are meant to grow old with strength, health, grace, and dignity. You do not have to be afraid of aging. You are meant to be able to wrestle with your grandkids and go for long walks with your friends and family. Growing older should be a wonderful, joyous process; it's not something to be dreaded and feared.

The majority of information in this book has been well-researched and applied to learning disabilities, brain development, and brain rehabilitation. This book is an extrapolation from this research combined with the "what ifs" of thoughts, observations, and experiences. After fourteen years of teaching this and witnessing the power of these movements, I can unequivocally tell you that the body is designed to heal, to move towards strength and health. I can also tell you that as the body heals, the whole person heals in their bodies and their souls.

Again, you are indeed awesomely and wonderfully made, always. Refuse to settle for any thought or belief that says less than this.

The Steel Geezer

"I am what they call a high miler. I'm 68, but if my life had an odometer, it would read in Roman Numerals. I qualify for two artificial knees, and until I found Original Strength, my rotator cuffs were rotator puffs. However, even if you combined these factors along with the lifelong back issues from heavy deadlifts and squats, one stroke, and a 5th heart attack that literally killed me, resulting in an Implantable Cardiac Defibrillator that looks like a can of sardines sticking out of my chest, everything was copacetic. OK, it was like, "Other than that, Mrs. Lincoln, how was the theater?"

To be honest, I've faced death so many times the hairs on the back of my neck don't stand up anymore. The death angel doesn't even bother showing up now; he figures it's just another false alarm. Besides, he knows I'm doing Original Strength.

How I discovered Tim Anderson and Original Strength could be summed up in just two words: **divine intervention**.

I have friends, family, medical records, a Sports Medicine Doctor, x-rays, and a personal physician who will tell you the wonders that have taken place since I started Pressing RESET. I can do dips, chins, push-ups, squats, and the whole enchilada—all pain-free. Heck, I can even give myself a black eye with my knee if I get carried away doing my standing cross crawls, and I couldn't even kick the cat before.

The Pressing RESET method is principle-based. I learned about principles 14 years ago from a gentleman who is a combat tactics special ops instructor. My eyes were opened to the wondrous possibilities of a principle-integrated life.

I learned that principles are immutable laws of universal reality. They are foundational, not mere techniques, tactics, procedures, or opinions. They are applicable across the entire spectrum of human function: physically, mentally, and spiritually. For this reason, there are no concerns regarding retention, as these principles are already embedded in your human hard drive. You do not acquire their benefits; ***they are yours by right****.*

The principles of Pressing RESET are simple and easy to integrate. They work for anyone and everyone, enabling you to experience your inherent right to healing, resilience, and the special, no-holds-barred life you are here to live.

Original Strength, endorsed by the Universe. Thanks, Tim."

—Freddie Mitchell, aka The Steel Geezer
Vancouver Island

LIFE STARTS WITH MOVEMENT

Babies develop ideally through learning how to move. Even before a child sees the light of this world, he starts developing his brain inside his mother's womb through movement. Once the child is born, the reflexes and movement patterns already etched deep inside his brain and spinal cord start building a fantastic foundation of reflexive strength through movement. These wonderful movement patterns that build reflexive strength enable more movements, and these more complex movements help develop the brain and nervous system. The very movements creating a child's strength further develop his nervous system. In other words, our body and brain are developed through a cycle of movement. The more we move through our natural movement patterns, the more we develop our brain. The more we develop our brain, the more efficient we become at moving. The more efficient we become at moving, the better we move and the more we further build our brain. This cycle can and should go on and on throughout our entire lives.

In case the above paragraph was confusing, here is a summation: When we were children, we learned to move through specific movement patterns etched deep inside our nervous system. Moving through these patterns, we developed and strengthened our body and brain. Brain development and body development are not mutually exclusive events. They go hand in hand. As one develops, the other is nourished and developed. Learning to move and engaging in movement even develops who we are as individuals. In *The Well Balanced Child*, Ewout Van-Manen points out, *"… physical movement is the basis for cognitive, social and emotional development."*[4] Let's look at the converse of Van-Manen's statement: A lack of cognitive, social, and emotional development can be traced back to a lack of physical movement.

The brain and the body nourish and develop each other. However, movement is the catalyst for this nourishment. Movement builds **everything** about you. Through movement, we create our "body map," our sense of self in space. This is called proprioception.[5] Our body is filled with sensors and proprioceptors in our skin, joints, tendons, fascia, and muscles that feed our brain with a sense of self every time we move and experience our environment. The more we move, the more we flood our brain with information from our proprioceptors about what our body is doing and where our body is at. This flood of information creates a "body map" or "movement map" in our brain. The better our body map is, the better we move.

Not only does movement improve your proprioception, it actually physically changes and improves your brain! Physical activity develops brain tissue![6] Inside your brain, there are millions of nerve connections, or neural networks. Movement improves the communication between these connections and actually cements new connections.[7] This is called neuroplasticity. Neuroplasticity is defined as the brain's ability to change and adapt its structure and function throughout life; this never stops! So, the more you move, and the better you move, the more complex and efficient your brain becomes. **The more complex and efficient your brain becomes, the better you move.**

Again, brain development and body development go hand in hand. It's a two-way street, and movement is the vehicle. Movement is the key to every facet of our health. It shapes everything about us: Our brains, our bodies, who we are as people, our emotions, our hormones, and even our mental health.[8]

Clearly, we were designed to move. Yet, most of us do not live in this design. Instead, many of us live static, sedentary lives. So over time, we lose our movement patterns because we replace them with sitting or being still. Through being sedentary, we slow our brain development or reverse it. Neuroplasticity works both ways. The brain can build new neural connections and the brain can remove unused neural connections. This process is called neuronal fitness or neuronal pruning.[9] Just as movement can shape and develop our brains, not moving can also shape and stunt the development of our brains

Simply put, for our brains to remain energy efficient they prune out the neural connections we don't need or the ones we don't use often. The neural connections in the brain represent what happens in the body. What we don't use, we lose. If we don't move, we lose the neural connections for our movements, meaning we also lose the ability to move well. And, if we don't move, we don't just lose those neural connections, we also lose the structures that enabled and facilitated those connections; we lose muscle, bone, joint, and structural integrity. Grab hold of this one thing: **Movement creates us.**

Movement creates us.

Today, we live in a world filled with technological innovations and conveniences. We have computers, cars, and the Internet. There is not much need for us to get up and move. Even if we want to go grocery shopping, we only have to jump online and click a button or two. Anything we want can be brought to us in a manner of minutes, and all we have to do is lift a finger. Do you remember malls? They are disappearing. This means the "mall walkers" are disappearing, too. More and more, we move less and less.

We are "growing" further away from having physical bodies capable of anything and toward having bodies capable of little more than holding chairs down. This is not the path we want to take.

We are wonderfully made, yet we don't allow ourselves to participate in the wonder for which we were created. Instead of moving anywhere and everywhere, most of us spend our time moving nowhere. We occupy the same square footage of a chair for hours and hours every day. Many kids today are being held captive by "smart" devices like phones and tablets. They are not going outside to play, they are not learning how to socialize and read physical cues from others. As a result they are not learning or building their movement repertoire, the very thing that will help them learn, communicate, create, and become emotionally mature. They are not even learning how to run, how to skip, or how to climb. Instead, they are learning how to live with anxiety, depression, and even diseases they were never meant to have. The point is we are getting further and further away from our design. We were made to move - and through movement, we are meant to live extraordinary lives. Movement *is* life to us.

A Season of Restoration

"I just completed reading your book. I have a history of back issues and dislocation of my Sacroiliac joint on the right side. I have managed these inconveniences with a consistent combination of yoga, running, strength training, seriously limiting time spent sitting, and PT when needed. Having seen few, if any, positive outcomes with surgical or pain medication intervention, I have avoided those avenues.

I recently have experienced rather uncomfortable levels of pain related to the sacral issue. After reading the cross-crawl, crawling, rocking and rolling instructions, I went to my mat and did all of these. Let me just say, the pain relief is miraculous! I am moving more fluidly and with no pain or stiffness after sitting. This is after one short session.

This technique seems to have reset the pelvis better than the bridge exercise prescribed by my physical therapist. What an amazing difference. I had a pain free night of sleep for the first time in many months. I cannot tell you how excited I am!"

My Best Wishes,
Sharon Steedly

THE X IS IN YOU

The road, or the map, to regaining our original strength revolves around the center of the X. The X is your body. And the center of your X, is your midsection, your "core." Having a reflexively strong and solid center is the key to regaining your original strength. Without a solid center, you will never be able to experience your full strength potential.

Please understand, a reflexively strong center is not something you can get from doing traditional abdominal exercises. It is built by engaging in your original movement patterns. These developmental movement patterns establish, stimulate, sharpen, and fortify your reflexive strength.

In truth, a solid center is developed through the global input (afferent information) from the entire body. It's the simplest of things, really, that contribute to making one resilient. Our ability to express any quality or anything at all is dependent on the information we generate and receive through our body. In the nervous system, information determines expression. Diaphragmatic breathing, engaging in developmental movement patterns, controlling the movements of the head, stimulating the skin, even the way we think—all of these sources of information, and more, contribute to the building a powerful center, thus allowing the expression of a powerful body.

You already know this but you are a fully integrated being. Everything about you works together to make your whole body powerful and strong. If you were to remove any one facet of your body (like robbing your feet's ability to feel by wearing thick soled shoes all of your life), or if you tried to isolate one of your body's many systems from the others, you would weaken your entire structure (your body). A child develops an amazingly strong and resilient body by fully integrating and weaving its whole being together through movement. An adult can do the same thing. You can restore your strong center, you can rebuild your X, by engaging in and exploring the same movements you did as a developing child.

Again, you are an X. In fact, you're an interwoven and layered series of Xs. Not only are you shaped like one big X, but everything about your inner workings is an X. Just look at an anatomy chart of muscles and notice how the muscles and tendons lie in relationship to one another. Even your DNA is in the shape of a double helix, a spiraling X. The body is literally a series of connected Xs from head to toe.

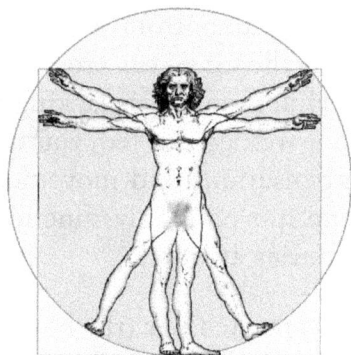

Leonardo da Vinci—Vitruvian Man
Public Domain Image

Can you see the X?

This is the drawing that inspired this chapter.

Draw a couple of diameter lines through any part of the circle. They cross at the man's navel. His navel is in the absolute center of the circle. The center is the secret to strength.

You also move in an "X-like" fashion. You are a contra-lateral moving being. At least you should be. When you walk, your left arm should match the swing of your right leg, and your right arm should match the swing of your left leg. Every step you take should be a fluid, coordinated motion causing your opposing shoulders to mirror your opposing hips.

Wildest of all, your nervous system is wired to receive and express information through your movements in an "X-like" fashion. The right side of your brain controls the left side of your body and the left side of your brain controls the right side of your body. And, the right side of your body feeds information to the left side of your brain and the left side of your body feeds information to the right side of your brain. Everything about you is an X.

Do you like apples? How do you like them criss-cross apple sauces?

Is the Force Strong Within You?

In order for you to be as strong and resilient as you were meant to be, the center of your X must be knit together properly. Your center, your core, is where the forces you generate from movements like crawling, walking, and throwing cross over from one side of your body to the other. These forces cross through your center from left to right, right to left, bottom to top, and top to bottom. The more "connected" your X is, the more efficiently the forces can cross over. You are made to be efficient and powerful. If your X is lacking in reflexive strength and your center is not well connected, you will have energy leakages that cause compensations and movement dysfunctions. These compensations and movement dysfunctions often result in weakness at best and injuries at worst.

Think of your core as the area from your pelvic floor (the bottom of your bottom) to the base of your neck with your belly button being in the dead center. However you think of the core, it is the crossroads of force production. When everything is working as it should, the core is the crossroads of efficient and powerful forces—the key to a strong and resilient body.[10] When things in the core are not functioning properly, the core can become the crossroads of energy chaos; forces end up going in areas they shouldn't go, creating unnecessary stresses, energy leakages, and movement dysfunctions. In other words, if your reflexive center, your reflexive core, is not functioning properly, you will not be as powerful or as resilient as you were meant to be, and you may be at a higher risk of injury, as well as a myriad of other issues like poor digestion, unbalanced hormones, sluggish metabolism and so on.

Baseballs and Wiffle Balls

To understand the importance of a solid center, look at the difference between baseballs and wiffle balls. A baseball is durable. Babe Ruth could hit a home run with the same baseball 100 times. As long as he never lost the baseball, he would be able to hit that same ball over and over again. Why? Because the baseball is solid. It has a solid center. The forces coming from Babe's powerful swing travel through the center of the ball, and the ball travels outside the park. After a while, the stitching may start to give way, and the cover may begin to unravel, but the ball is still a ball, and Babe could still play with it. The baseballs are remarkably resilient. Because they are solid, they can absorb and transfer large amounts of energy repeatedly without becoming damaged.

Wiffle balls, on the other hand, are not so durable. Babe Ruth could hit a wiffle ball, and it may only travel as far as second base. It would not even come close to making it outside of the ballpark. And, if he were lucky, The Babe may get one more hit out of the wiffle ball before it cracked or split. Why? Wiffle balls are hollow, they have no center. The forces coming from Babe's powerful swing would travel around the shell of the wiffle ball. These forces would ultimately be too great for the shell to remain intact, causing it to split. Wiffle balls are pretty fragile when it comes to absorbing and transferring energy. They can survive the hits of small children but can't withstand the mighty blows of a well-connected adult.

In this analogy, we were created to be more like baseballs, not wiffle balls. The human body needs a solid center to effectively mitigate and transfer all the forces it generates and all the other forces it receives from life (think of life as a baseball bat).

Did you know that the human body produces 2 times its weight in force when you walk, in every single step you take? If you weighed only 100 pounds, you would be producing 200 pounds of force with every step you made. When you run, you generate 6 to 8 times your weight in force. When you sprint, you generate ten to twelve times your weight in force! For a 100 pound person, that would be 1000 pounds of force generated with every single step made while sprinting! How many people do you know who only weigh 100 pounds?

You might think you don't even know anyone who sprints, but you should, and it is sad if you don't. But can you see why your X must have a solid center? Those powerful forces we generate and encounter should travel efficiently and appropriately through our bodies. If we have a "hollow" center and our X is not adequately woven together, we could become quite fragile like the wiffle ball.

The baseball and wiffle ball analogy may be overly simplistic, but hopefully, it conveys the importance of having a durable, solid center. Your body was created to last and withstand the ravages of time and life. You are even meant to be more durable than a baseball!

You Are Fully Integrated

Remember, your body is fully integrated. Your X is knit together by everything about you. Your head movement is tied to your core.[11] Your grip is tied to your core. Your feet are tied to your core. Your skin is tied to your core. Your emotions are even tied to your core. Your core is tied to **EVERYTHING**. Your entire body is interconnected and this interconnection is what solidifies your center. Isn't this fascinating? Nothing about you is isolated from any other part of you. **Everything about you is integrated into the whole of you.** Your body was created to be in perfect union with itself.

Unfortunately, we are really good at not honoring our design. We've created conveniences in life that allow us to be comfortable so we don't have to move. Things like chairs, rearview mirrors, computers, remote controls (children!), smart phones, etc. We have become really good at not moving our heads or our bodies. Therefore, we have become masters of dis-integration. As a result, we start unraveling. We lose some of our movement patterns, we stagnate our vestibular system (we dull or lose our balance), we lose our reflexively stable core, and we become broken. We lose these things not simply because we do not use them, but because we do not need them with our current lifestyles.

> Everything about you is integrated into the whole of you.

Fortunately, we can Press RESET, weave our centers together again, and regain our original strength. **To become physically resilient and strong again, we must do what we did as babies: build our stability and mobility through movement.**

A long, long time ago, in a diaper far, far away, you developed your strength and resiliency through a series of specific movements. Movements we call RESETS. These RESETS are just that: resets. When we reengage in these movements, we Press RESET on our bodies, and our strength is reborn.

Connecting The X

"I've gotten tremendous results when I put crawling into serious practice. Not only have I increased my strength, endurance and flexibility but I think I have found the most important thing: freedom. If you are familiar with some Systema Martial Arts practitioners (if not check on YouTube), you can see that they are moving with grace and power. I discovered this grace and power from doing the OS RESETS, not only from crawling. By the way, Systema is based on breathing, another wonderful concept from OS.

Now, I am not an emotional slave to the other tools and training methods. Now, everything has become the tool! A rock, table, stairs, a bench, the floor, I can use and train with everything! This is freedom. I can move my body in all positions and directions with grace and I don't worry about injuries. I have true resilience and freedom. So crawling is much more than a strength and conditioning tool for me. I will always recommend the OS RESETS to people around me, because I know the power behind those 'silly' moves. I am not a believer anymore, I just know as I have experienced this to be true in my life. Even if I do get an injury, I have confidence because I know the OS RESETS."

—Łukasz (Luke)
Poland

PRESSING RESET

Have you ever been frustrated with your computer or "smart" phone because it froze up on you or didn't seem to be working correctly? What did you do? More than likely, you performed a reset on it, or you rebooted it. Usually, this resolves our issue. Resetting our technological devices has been the saving grace that has saved nearly all of us from weeping and gnashing our teeth. For whatever reason, performing a reset seems to return them to proper working order magically. When we reset our devices, the operating system gets refreshed, and all the programs on top of it begin working properly; order and peace are restored to our world.

What if you could reset your body in the same way? What if you could not move the way you knew you should be able to move, or you weren't as strong as you knew you should be? What if you could simply press a button, reset your body's operating system, and restore your optimal potential?

You can!

Engaging in the same developmental movements you made as a child, the movements preprogrammed into your nervous system, is like pressing a reset button on your body. That's really what this book is about: five developmental movement patterns. We call these movement patterns RESETS. Engaging in any one or all of these RESETS refreshes our nervous systems, allowing our bodies to respond by functioning optionally and in proper working order.

How does this happen? "Pressing RESET" refreshes the nervous system by providing clear and "safe" information to the brain. This prompts the brain to supply better information back to the body, establishing and restoring the proper reflexive connections throughout the body. In other words, Pressing RESET improves the afferent information going to the brain which in turn improves the efferent information going back to the body. This improved exchange of information restores the body's *reflexive strength*.

Reflexive strength is the foundation of movement expression. It is the combination, or union, of reflexive stability, reflexive mobility, and reflexive control.

Really, reflexive strength is the body's ability to anticipate and respond to movement before and as it happens. It is predictive and reactive strength. It is automatic, non-cognitive strength. It's the strength that protects us and preserves us. Always. At least it should be.

The more reflexive strength we have, the more we can express movement and participate in all the incredible adventures, experiences, hobbies, and skills we want to enjoy in life.

> Reflexive strength is the body's ability to anticipate and respond to movement before and as it happens.

Without reflexive strength, obtaining the skill needed to achieve your objective would be impossible. When we do not have all of our reflexive stability, mobility, or control, we do not have our full reflexive strength. We cannot fully express all the mobility, strength, power, speed, and fluidity we were designed to express. If we cannot express ourselves optimally, we are limited and forced to live diminished lives. I would even argue that without our reflexive strength fully intact, fulfilling our purpose in life would be challenging.

Just know that your reflexive strength is your foundation for expression and is a culmination of everything about you.

In the medical model, the body is often viewed as compartments and separate parts. For example, mobility is viewed as a separate quality from stability or strength. Mobility was never meant to be segregated from stability or strength, and that is certainly not how the body develops or operates. The truth is that strength, stability, and mobility are all components of the same thing: movement or the control of movement.

For example, when a child learns how to lift its very large head, it is building stability, strength, control, AND mobility at the same time. Yes, babies are born mobile, but they are like rag dolls; they cannot control their mobility. It is only when they build the strength and stability to move and hold their heads on the horizon that they also develop the *control* of their mobility. If any one of these qualities is lacking, they are all lacking. They are all designed to be built together, in unison with one another as they combine together as expression.

Stability, mobility, control and strength are all parts of the whole. They are the two sides of the coin or the four sides of the same square. For example, if a man lacks the mobility to be able to touch his toes, more than likely it is because he lacks the reflexive stability in his core to stabilize his spine. The brain is smart. If the body's stabilizers, the muscles that stabilize joints, are not working correctly, the brain turns prime movers, the muscles that move joints, into stabilizers. When prime movers become stabilizers, they can no longer move the body the way they were intended and the mobility of the body becomes limited. When mobility is limited, strength is limited. Thus the body cannot optimally express its full potential for mobility, stability, or control because the overall movement expression—*reflexive strength*—is limited.

When we Press RESET and engage in our original movement template, we begin to restore and regain our reflexive strength, our foundation—we restore our reflexive stability, mobility, and control. They are all parts of the same expression and they are all governed by our reflexes. This is the foundation that our strength, health and resiliency are built upon. **In order to become as healthy and resilient as possible, we have to own our reflexive strength.** We do this by Pressing RESET often in order to deepen our "roots" and establish a foundation of reflexive strength. By Pressing RESET consistently we are constantly reinforcing and nurturing our reflexive strength throughout our lifetime.

Perhaps the most wonderful thing about Pressing RESET is that you don't have to understand how your body works in order to do it. You don't have to have a firm grasp on your neurology, your physiology, or your biology. You don't even have to know the Latin names of your muscles. All you have to do is engage in your design. And your design is to move in specific ways or patterns. You came into the world with these movement patterns and therefore you cannot ever lose these movement patterns. They "came with the frame" *so to speak*. When you engage in these patterns, GOOD things happen.

> In order to become as healthy and resilient as possible, we have to own our reflexive strength.

The Big Five RESETS

There are five developmental movement patterns we call RESETS. Engaging in these movement patterns refreshes the central nervous system and it restores and "sharpens" the reflexive neuromuscular connections throughout the body. Consistently engaging in these movement patterns and their variations embeds, myelinates, these neural connections making them very energy efficient and ready for use. The result of having these efficient, "sharp," neural connections is they allow the body and mind to be capable of reaching and expressing their full potential in both movement and thought. This is how we can restore our original strength!

Original Strength's Big Five RESETS:

1. Proper Diaphragmatic Breathing
2. Head Movements
3. Rolling
4. Rocking
5. Crawling/Cross-crawling/Gait pattern

In the chapters that follow, we shall explore the details of each of these RESETS. But before we do that, let's take a look at the ONLY rules inside of our method. We emphasize the word "only" here because when it comes to Pressing RESET, there is no algorithm and the best thing we can do is honor a person's body and "start where they are."

In this book we are presenting these movement patterns in the order they appear through the developmental sequence, but when it comes to Pressing RESET you need not move through the RESETS in a specific order. They are all great for you, but there is no magic order or complex reps and sets scheme that must be followed. The magic happens when you do them, all of them or some of them, or even one of them. And that's about as complicated as it gets.

Actually, it's pretty simple. When we engage in the original movement patterns of our developmental sequence, we are basically honoring the 3 pillars of being a human. When we honor these pillars, we are Pressing RESET on our bodies.

The 3 Pillars of Human *Being*

"...A cord of 3 strands is not quickly broken."
—Ecclesiastes 4:12

There are 3 pillars of human being, 3 foundational "movements" or practices we were created to do continually throughout our lives. If we are doing these 3 things, we are essentially always Pressing RESET. These 3 pillars are embedded inside of the developmental sequence (the Big 5 RESETS):

1. Breathe the way you were designed to breathe, the way you did when you were born - Close your lips, rest your tongue against the roof of your mouth, and breathe in and out through your nose.
2. Activate your vestibular system - Move your eyes, head and body often. Return your eyes and head to the horizon often.
3. Engage in your gait pattern, your contra-lateral movement patterns (like crawling, walking, skipping, running) often.

These are the 3 pillars of human *being*. If you do these 3 things, you will return to your original design and become as strong and healthy as you could ever hope to be, as you were meant to be.

The Hope in Movement

"I was diagnosed with ALS fifteen years ago. It's a disease that robs the muscles of their motor neurons; resulting in limited movement. Since my personal goal was to keep my body active and moving for as long as possible, I had to learn "how" to move all over again—from the ground up! Incorporating the Original Strength RESETS into my daily exercise has helped me both regain and retain my body's fundamental movement patterns. In fact, all the Original Strength information and exercises are informative and helpful. I learned how to maintain my core strength, joint mobility, sense of balance and have a positive attitude. Fifteen years after my diagnosis, I am moving on!"

–Dagmar Munn
Arizona

The Breath of Life

Proper breathing is vital to health, strength, and resiliency. If you are not currently breathing properly, relearning how to breathe could be the most critical seed in this entire book. Breathing is perhaps the most overlooked and undervalued reflex you possess.

When a child is born, breathing is the first real reflex and movement they engage in. Babies breathe correctly right from the start. They breathe in and out of their nose and fully use their diaphragm to fill their lungs. Babies don't breathe up in their neck and chest like most adults do. A child pulls air into the bottom of their lungs with their diaphragm. They breathe in their design, and this is the beginning of strength.

Breathing is not simply a mechanism for exchanging oxygen and carbon dioxide. It is also a vehicle for obtaining unlimited strength potential; it removes all barriers to physical expression. Sometimes, things are hidden from us in plain sight. When children are breathing, they are not merely "breathing"; they are building their brains, strengthening their bodies, and providing a base of "support" to regulate their emotions. We see their bodies move on the outside, but who could have ever dreamed what was happening on the inside?

Breath is life in the fullest sense of the word life. If that sounds strange or even crazy, know that breathing affects every facet of your entire being. **Breathing can even affect how your genes express themselves.**[12] This is why it is so crucial that you breathe the way you were created to breathe.

Adults unlearn or compensate for this natural breathing reflex for various reasons. Through trauma, fear, or any number of other reasons, many adults trade "belly breathing" (diaphragmatic breathing) for shallow "chest breathing." In doing so, they weaken their core, the center of their X. Worse than that, they send a clear message to their brains: "I am not safe." Over time, this repeated message of being in danger alters the entire body's well-being.

If this is you, if you are a chest breather, relearning and regaining your natural way of breathing can be the greatest step you ever take towards regaining your original strength. In fact, it may be impossible to unlock your full strength and health potential without breathing properly. All your attempts to become healthy and resilient will be undermined by a faulty breathing pattern—a faulty foundation of fear, stress, and weakness.

Just in case you don't remember when you were born, you were a diaphragmatic nasal breather - you were a "belly breather" who breathed almost exclusively in and out through your nose. Just watch any newborn baby, and you will see their little bellies rise up and down when they breathe. They are taking full advantage of their lung volume by effortlessly breathing with their diaphragm (let's call it the "breathing muscle"). They are also strengthening their diaphragm by breathing through their small nasal passages. When a child breathes, the diaphragm pulls a vacuum in the lungs, allowing them to fill themselves with life-giving air. Diaphragmatic breathing also moves and massages the internal organs, improving their function and aiding digestion. And perhaps most surprisingly, the diaphragm works with the pelvic floor and other muscles surrounding your spine to help create a reflexively stable, strong center. This is our foundation for strength and power. We establish this foundation through breath.

It may help to think of your diaphragm as the "captain" of your inner core musculature, the center of your center. When you breathe with the diaphragm, your diaphragm works in unison with these inner core muscles, providing reflexive stability and protection for your spine. In a way, your diaphragm is like the ceiling of your center, and your pelvic floor is like the floor of your center. These two move and work together when you breathe to form a "cylinder of strength" in your core. The stronger this cylinder is, the more strength, power, speed, and resilience you will possess.

Again, you were born breathing properly with your diaphragm. But life happens. Most people end up employing compensatory breathing patterns by using their accessory breathing muscles, their emergency breathing muscles. These are the muscles in the rib cage, neck, and shoulders. The accessory breathing muscles are the muscles a baby uses when breathing is compromised and in distress. When babies use these muscles to breathe, they are usually sick and need emergency medical attention. Our accessory/emergency breathing muscles are intended to help us during an emergency. They are helpful in helping us run away from danger or fight against it. But after the danger passes, we are supposed to return to our default breathing design.

Many of us become "neck and chest breathers" for fear-based reasons. We use our emergency breathing muscles to breathe twenty-four hours a day, seven days a week. We then get stuck in a perpetual web of danger that leads to weakness, sickness, and frailty.

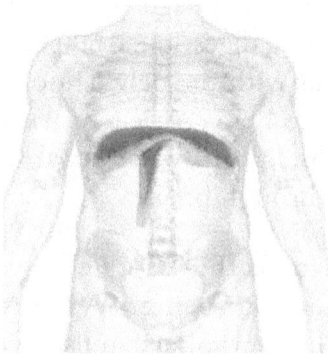

This is what the diaphragm muscle looks like. It is this muscle that truly makes you resilient.

And like most muscles, the diaphragm can be trained. It can grow stronger and efficient with use!

In my own life, I am fairly certain I know exactly when I started using my emergency breathing muscles and overrode my default breathing pattern. It was when I was in middle school. I was a scrawny kid, and as you probably know, middle school can be a harsh world for insecure teenagers. I didn't want to get picked on, beat up, or singled out, so I started sucking in my gut and puffing out my chest. Like a proud peacock, I was trying to look much bigger than I was. It didn't work! I still got picked on, so I started lifting weights and continued my new practice of being a chest breather. I got pretty good at it. The stress of middle school and the fear of being the weakest in the herd were strong enough to make me override my natural breathing pattern. It can start as simple as that for anyone. There is a potential lesson here: cognitively holding a posture to look stronger can make you weaker.

Again, we do have accessory respiratory muscles for a reason; they are our emergency breathing muscles. They are reserved for emergencies or times of extreme stress when we need more air. But we shouldn't need to use these breathing muscles all the time, especially while we are being sedentary. They are our fight-or-flight breathing muscles intended to help us survive the threats of calamity. In the absence of an emergency, we should not be using these accessory breathing muscles. Chronically breathing with these emergency breathing muscles sends a consistent message of fear to the brain and this can cause a myriad of unwanted issues throughout the body.

Danger, Danger!

Every breath you take sends one of two messages to your brain:

1. I am safe.
2. I am not safe.

When you breathe with your lips shut, your tongue resting on the roof of your mouth, and your diaphragm pulling air into the bottom of your lungs, you are sending the message, "I am safe." This helps you live in your parasympathetic state, your rest and digest state, where all is well, and your body is likely functioning optimally. You could even call this state your Thrive state. In this state, life feels GOOD.

When you breathe through your mouth, your tongue isn't resting on the roof of your mouth, and you use your accessory breathing muscles, filling mostly the top portion of your lungs, you are sending the message, "I am not safe." This causes you to live in your sympathetic state, your fight or flight state, where, over time, things start to "fly off the rails." You could call this state your Survival state. Living in this state is where stress accumulates in the body, anxiety takes hold, muscles hold tension, hormones become unbalanced, inflammation sets in, body systems become compromised, digestion gets subpar, sleep is disrupted, and frailness and illness settle in. In this state, life feels BLAH.

Living in survival mode, constantly telling your brain that you're not safe with how you are breathing, starts to unravel the whole tapestry of your being. For example, living and breathing in "emergency mode" leads to postural issues and muscular compensations that affect the entire body. Mouth and accessory breathing leads to forward head carriage, neck pain, poor thoracic mobility, and kyphosis (a hunched, slouched forward posture). Worse still, it can cause a loss of reflexive strength (stability) in the body's core muscles.

Remember, when we don't have our reflexive strength, we become fragile, not just physically but also in our minds and emotions. A strong, capable body leads to confidence and a general state of well-being. A weak, fragile body leads to insecurity and self-absorption. Dysfunctional breathing, "I am not safe" breathing, can lead to a lifetime of walking on eggshells and feeling vulnerable. It can wreck everything about you.

Many people spend a lifetime breathing like this. Are you one of them? Be aware of how you breathe and ensure you are breathing in your design. This is so important on many levels, especially when considering how your breathing ultimately affects how you interact with and experience the world.

And that's good news! We can change our world at the speed of our nervous system by changing the way we breathe. If we can change our breathing pattern *for the bad*, then we can also retrain our breathing pattern and change it back *for the good*. Breathing is a natural subconscious reflex (like all reflexes). However, this subconscious reflex can also be adjusted through awareness and conscious training or effort. If practiced enough, over time, we can revert to our default way of breathing, where the default way becomes subconscious again.

This is made possible through neuroplasticity. We create the patterns, movements, thoughts, and neural connections we want our brain to flourish in through accumulating repetitions via regular practice and engagement. Consciously and consistently practicing our original pattern for breath tips the scales in our favor and cements this desired pattern in our brain. It also robs and weakens the other dysfunctional breathing pattern we want to replace. In the end, consciously engaging in our original breathing pattern relays the message to our brain: "I am safe." This is the message of growth and flourishing. It leads to vitality.

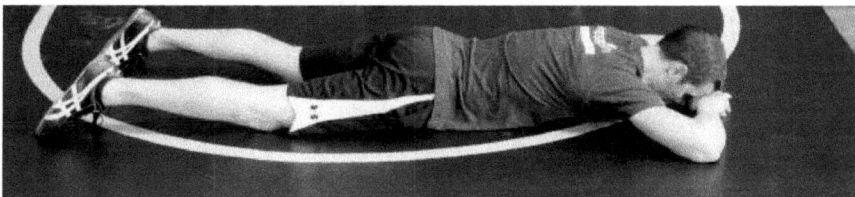

In the *Pressing RESET* courses, we introduce crocodile breathing as one way to relearn and rediscover how to breathe functionally. In crocodile breathing, you lie on your belly and rest your forehead on the back of your hands. While inhaling through your nose and keeping your tongue on the roof of your mouth, try to breathe down into your belly. If you do this correctly, you will feel your belly will push against the floor. This will cause your lower back to rise up and down as you breathe. This is such a fantastic and gentle way to mobilize your lower back. In fact, this way of breathing often resolves lower back pains and issues.

When crocodile breathing, the belly does not just push into the floor, the sides of your belly will also expand and get wider, just like a crocodile!

This is an important fact about our design to breathe - "belly breathing" is not just simply allowing movement at the belly. True breath is three-dimensional; it's a 360° motion where the body's center expands in all directions as the breath enters the lungs. Oftentimes, people only focus on the belly when trying to relearn how to breathe. They establish another dysfunctional breathing pattern by limiting and constricting the diaphragm and other accessory breathing muscles from functioning fully. The entire cylinder should expand with breath, not just the front. When you practice breathing, relax your center and let it move in every direction.

Again, crocodile breathing is just one way and one position to rediscover breath. There are many ways to practice belly breathing. Our courses cover a series of breathing "regressions" that help most people rediscover the magic of breathing and its correlation to better health, movement, and performance.

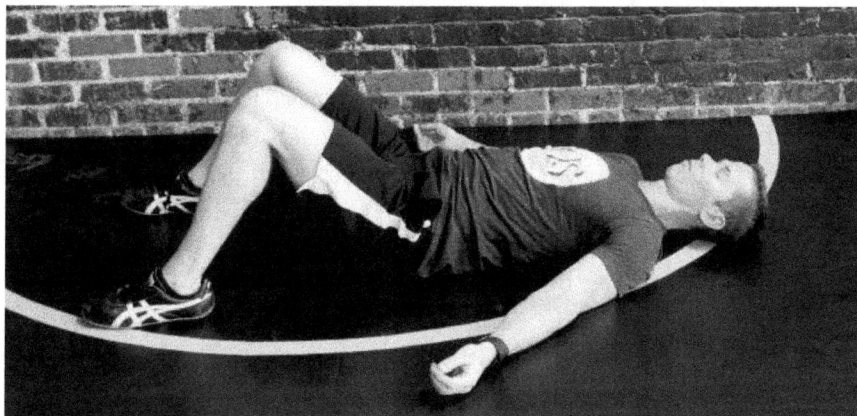

This position is a favorite in group sessions at the Original Strength Institute. Look, it even puts Tim to sleep...

Perhaps the most effective way to remember how to breathe is to just spend time on the floor like a child and deliberately try to breathe into your belly while you explore different positions. You will likely find that some positions make it very easy to find your diaphragm while others make it more challenging. I encourage you to dive into the positions that make it easy; these positions will help you accumulate those restoring repetitions. The easier positions will also lend themselves to the more challenging positions later.

Some of you may need to look beyond a position to find your breath. You may also need extra tactile information to help your brain "find" your diaphragm. For example, you may need to rest your hands or place a light weight (like a 3-5 pound sandbag) on your belly to increase awareness of that area. Or, it may help to blow out all the air you can possibly blow out and then "let go" and allow the air to rush back into your lungs. This is often a surefire way to discover your diaphragm again and learn what it feels like for air to fill the bottom of your lungs.

In the beginning, we are looking for positions and sensations that allow us to remember how to breathe in our design. Ultimately, we want to be able to breathe in our design in every position, activity, and situation we encounter. Whether it be running a marathon, strength training, or having a crucial conversation with a colleague or adversary, we want to breathe and flourish through the default message of our breath: "I am safe." This is where we will be able to express our full potential in every way possible.

So, it doesn't matter how you rediscover your breath as long as you can rediscover it. Relearn how to breathe: Close your lips, keep your tongue on the roof of your mouth, breathe in and out of your nose, and expand your cylinder in all directions.

Note: At the risk of being redundant, "Belly breathing" simply means relaxing your center and allowing it to expand in all directions as your diaphragm descends to fill your lungs. **The rib cage can and should still expand with your breath.** We are not trying to isolate movement in the belly and inhibit the rib cage from moving. We are simply trying to naturally fill our lungs from the bottom to the top, from the back to the front, and everywhere in between. To do this, we need to relax our belly and allow natural movement of the rib cage. Don't overthink it. Try the above tips and rediscover your breath. It's one of the most important time investments you could ever make.

Hold Your Tongue

While we are on the subject of breathing, let's talk about the tongue. You've likely noticed I've instructed you to rest your tongue on the roof of your mouth. Believe it or not, where you keep your tongue matters. In fact, it may be a critical detail to your overall health. Your tongue is designed to rest against the roof of your mouth, behind your front teeth. If you're unsure where this position is, swallow and feel where your tongue goes as you swallow. It should move up against the roof of your mouth. This is your tongue's "home position" and it is a HUGE RESET for your nervous system. We often call this position, or this action, the RESET within the RESETS.

Simply placing the tongue on the roof of the mouth encourages nasal breathing, and nasal breathing encourages diaphragmatic breathing. Yes, you can breathe diaphragmatically through your mouth, but you are designed to naturally breathe through your nose. After all, this is how we are able to smell things! It is worth noting that while breathing through the nasal passages is optimal, there are some people who may not be able to do so. Being tongue-tied or having restricted nasal passages because of issues like a broken nose or a deviated septum can make nasal breathing quite challenging. Knowing what I now know, I think overcoming the difficulty is worth the effort.

If you are able to breathe through your nasal passages, you should make every effort to do so. Not only does nasal breathing encourage our diaphragm to work properly, but it is also our first line of defense against bacteria and viruses that may be in the air. It also warms the air up before it enters our lungs, and it even adds nitric oxide to the air that we breathe in. Our sinus cavities create nitric oxide, which helps keep our brain, heart, and blood vessels healthy. When we breathe through our mouths, we are missing out on these "gifts" of our design.

Another benefit of breathing through the nose is it can literally make you stronger. Nasal passages are smaller than the opening of the mouth. Breathing in through these smaller, narrow passages helps create more intra-abdominal pressure between your diaphragm and pelvic floor. This increased intra-abdominal pressure helps you become stronger and more resilient by creating a "muscle girdle" through and around your center. This higher pressurized "muscle girdle" is built and maintained through the reflexive action of diaphragmatic breathing through the nasal passages.

Strength Starts Here

Breathing with your diaphragm, the way you were born breathing, is the beginning of strength. Strength in the human body is built in layers, and our breath establishes the epicenter. Moving through the phases of our developmental sequence wraps more and more layers of strength over that center. This is one of the many reasons why it is so important to breathe properly; we build strength from the center out.

Keep in mind that strength is not just a physical expression. We can also have strength in our minds and emotions. Proper breathing helps to establish a foundation for this type of strength. Remember, when a person is breathing properly, they are likely in "rest and digest mode" or "Thrive" mode. Diaphragmatic breathers have more peace and confidence. Their bodies and minds can rest, repair, and respond to life appropriately. Having peace of mind helps us to better regulate our emotions; it helps us to develop emotional maturity. This allows us to better cope with the stress of life.

There are always parallels of truth. If we build strength from the center, then our soul, mind, and emotions are at the core of our being. If our soul is resilient because it is at peace, our body will be able to express itself optimally. Consider this: You've never had a thought or an emotion that your body did not know about. Your thoughts and emotions are information that your brain is always searching and sifting through while asking one question: "Am I safe?"

If your thoughts and emotions are "not safe," your body will express this information in the form of tension, pain, weakness, or fear. These things weaken and inhibit our ability to express our strength, mobility, speed, and power. They also weaken our ability to express creativity, logic, and reasoning. It may seem wild, but how we breathe affects everything about us.

Every. Single. Thing.

Anyway, it's a two-way street. Your breath affects your soul; your soul affects your body. Strength comes from being able to live in a state of peace. Where the mind leads, the body will follow. If your thoughts are stressful and chaotic, your body will also reflect stress and chaos in your movements and your other bodily functions. If your thoughts are calm and fluid, your body will reflect your mind with calm and fluid movements. Life is not meant to be a constant emergency. Even if it was, we were created to overcome and mitigate the emergency through calm, steady strength—through breath! **Simply put, you can survive in the presence of fear, but you were made to thrive in the presence of peace.**

> Simply put, you can survive in the presence of fear, but you were made to thrive in the presence of peace.

It is vitally important you breathe the way you were designed to breathe. If you do not, you will never operate in the full capacity of your design. If this were the only thing you learned how to do from this book, it alone would be enough to change your life for the better. Your original strength, the foundation of you, starts with a breath. You owe it to yourself to remember how you were designed to breathe.

Breathe:

- Assume the desired position above.
- Keep your mouth closed.
- Place (rest) your tongue on the roof of your mouth. (If you're not sure exactly where this position is or how it should feel, just swallow, and your tongue will go there automatically.)
- Breathe in and out through your nose.

- Pull air deep down into your belly.
- Become strong!

To learn more, here is a playlist of breathing exercises:

https://youtube.com/playlist?list=PL9v3pv_KGM7v7yNiQJ hnHkf5WWDwv7cMn&si=BdzQNw2mKchz93EF

Take A Breath

"I have a client that had a chronic hip flexor problem and couldn't even pry himself with a crowbar into a squat. Once his breathing pattern changed from chest breathing to diaphragm breathing, he could now hang out in a rock-bottom squat for a time. This was the first time his pain went away in 5 years since a mountain bike accident which triggered his dysfunction."

Trevor Trebbien
Oregon

"Diaphragmatic breathing is great for movement but also has many other applications. In my work with students in the military, it's taught as 'tactical breathing.' We use it in teaching marksmanship. Tactical breathing can be used to slow the heart rate to make a precise long-distance shot, or it can help get accurate hits with a handgun.

We also teach students to use it to help control stress in many situations. I've had students successfully use it during some of our more stressful meetings and negotiation scenarios to calm themselves as things get tense. An example of how diaphragmatic breathing could be helpful in a stressful environment would be if you were standing, you might ask to have a seat. During that short time, you move to sit down; if you 'set your breathing,' it will help you gain some clarity, and you can refocus, mitigating your stress.

Just as with Pressing RESET, it may seem to be a small part of the process…but in reality, it's a vital root to the process. We believe in using diaphragmatic breathing in situations that could be life or death, national strategic-level success or failure, or just keeping a calm head."

Chad Faulkner
US Army

Move Your Head

The next RESET we will discuss involves learning how to control the movements of your head. Learning how to move the head and developing head control is how a child starts adding a layer of strength to the epicenter of strength created by breathing. For children, as well as for adults, mastering head control is essential to having balance, posture, and coordination.[13]

Look at that again: *mastering head control is essential to having balance, posture, and coordination.*

Another way to say this is that mastering head control is essential for having a healthy, happy life. Suppose we don't have good balance, posture, and coordination. In that case, we cannot fully enjoy our body's potential and, therefore, cannot fully navigate through life as well as we would want to. Our ability to control the movements of our head and activate our vestibular system is crucial to living life better.

The Vestibular System

Head control is so vital to your overall strength and health because your head is the home of your vestibular system (your balance system). Your vestibular system is a set of organs that reside behind your ears. These vestibular organs are highly sensitive movement detection organs called the utricle, saccule, and semicircular canals.[14] Without getting too scientific, they are like having your own internal gyroscopes inside your head. These organs are filled with tiny hairs and a gel-like substance. When your head moves, the liquid substance moves these tiny hairs and sends information to your brain. Your gyroscopes work to give you equilibrium and balance.[15] Their job is to keep your head level with the horizon.

Again, you have two of these gyroscope-like organs in your head, one behind each ear. These tiny little gyroscopes are what make you who you are. If they are functioning properly, your world is "right side up," and all is well with you.

Without a healthy vestibular system, you cannot have a healthy, strong body or be your best self. In fact, great health cannot exist separate from a healthy vestibular system. The vestibular system is perhaps the most important sensory system you have. Everything about you is shaped by how your vestibular system functions: Your sense of self, your reality, your balance, your posture, your ability to hold your head up and maintain your gaze on the horizon, your ability to learn, your experiences, everything.[16]

In truth, you want all your systems to function optimally. That probably never needs to be said. But you can function without other sensory systems and lead a somewhat "normal" life. For example, a blind man can learn to be independent and get around almost as well as people who have sight. In many ways, a blind man may learn how to enjoy life through other heightened senses that people with sight will not experience. However, a person with a compromised vestibular system may not be able to have a "normal" life.

Ask anyone who has ever had vertigo, and they will tell you how important a healthy vestibular system is for feeling "normal" and healthy. It is pretty hard to navigate through the world when your vestibular system can't tell which way is up or down, left or right, still or spinning, level or tilted. The vestibular system is your gravitational force, horizon level, and motion detection system. It is designed to constantly tell your brain where your head and body are about the earth.

VESTIBULAR SYSTEM

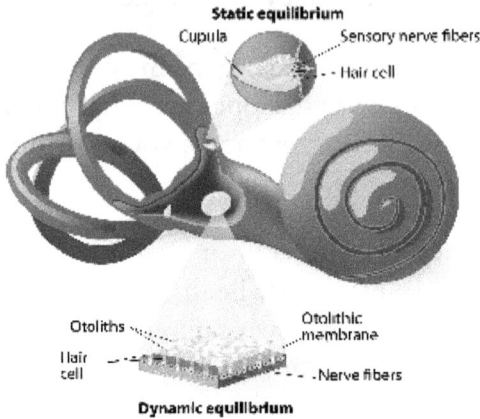

Static equilibrium
Cupula
Sensory nerve fibers
Hair cell

Otoliths
Otolithic membrane
Hair cell
Nerve fibers
Dynamic equilibrium

You have two of these in your head. One behind each ear. These tiny little gyroscopes are what make you who you are.

One of the reasons the vestibular system is one of, if not THE, most important sensory system you have is because it is the first sensory system to begin developing in the fetus, inside the mother's womb. It begins developing about 21 days after conception,[17] and it becomes fully developed about 5 months after conception.[18] This means 4 months before a child is born, he has a fully functioning vestibular system.

This fully functioning vestibular system detects every movement the mother makes. The mother's heartbeat, her breath, her laughs, when she walks, moves, sneezes, snores - all of this information is detected and travels through the child's vestibular system, helping to develop the child's brain.

Once the child is born, it encounters a greater pull of gravity. This new world of gravity and the head-righting reflex further stimulate the vestibular system. We are all born with a head-righting reflex. This reflex is designed to put our eyes and head on the horizon; it demands us to learn how to hold and move our head level with the horizon. The earth's gravitational pull and the head-righting reflex force the child to learn how to move and develop head control. This further shapes the child's brain and develops his nervous system.

Do you see the brilliance and wonder in the design? We are absolutely made to move, and the more we move, the more we become.

It's worth noting that the vestibular system is not just our balance system. It is also the foundation of all our other sensory systems. In fact, all of the information we sense (minus smell) and the movements we make get routed through the vestibular system before it enters the brain.[19]

Your vestibular system is the hub - the information crossroads - for all the information that goes into your brain. This information, combined with the information generated by the vestibular system itself, feeds and nourishes your brain and creates who you are.

This includes the information your proprioceptive system provides or your inner *sense of self*. The proprioceptive system is the collection of information about what your body is doing and what is going on around your body. It is intimately tied to your vestibular system.[20] Together, your proprioceptive and vestibular systems form your body map, or movement map, in your brain. The better your movement map is, the better you move.

Your visual system is also tied to your vestibular system. Ninety percent of the cells in your visual system respond to vestibular information.[21] Your autonomic nervous system (which controls the things you don't consciously control, like your heart rate, respiratory rate, digestion, perspiration, arousal, etc.) is also tied to your vestibular system.[22] Your vestibular system is also connected to every single muscle in your body, especially the core and neck muscles![23] Even your emotions are affected by your vestibular system.[24] Everything about you is connected to your vestibular system.

Everything.

Therefore, a healthy vestibular system is critical to having a healthy body and living a wonderful life.

How do you build a healthy vestibular system or repair a compromised one?

You honor its design. Your vestibular system is designed to detect movement and receive information. If you "feed" that design, you can improve its function. When you were a child, you fed the design by living in it and learning how to move. Today, as an adult, you can build a healthy vestibular system the same way: relearn how to move and then move often! The more you move, the more you stimulate your vestibular system. The more you stimulate your vestibular system, the more neural connections you make in your brain and your body. You can move your way towards a healthier vestibular system, thus having a healthier, stronger, more resilient body.

It has even been shown that children who receive regular vestibular stimulation show advanced motor skill development.[25] Remember, all your muscles are neurologically connected to your vestibular system. If you continually stimulate your vestibular system, you are essentially stimulating all of the muscles in your body, especially your core and neck muscles. Isn't that awesome?

Not only that but the more you stimulate and strengthen your vestibular system, the more you strengthen or solidify the health of all of your body's other systems. You are completely integrated. Improving any part of you improves the whole of you. Your vestibular system is not merely any part of you. It is a foundational part of you if not THE foundational part of you. You CANNOT function properly without it.

Consider this. If movement improves the vestibular system and heals the body, then not moving does just the opposite. When you don't move, you are not stimulating the vestibular system. In other words, you are not stimulating your brain, nervous system, or neuro-muscular connections. Think of it this way, everything about the body follows the rule, "use it or lose it." The vestibular system is no different. If we neglect our vestibular system by living a sedentary life, we ask it to deteriorate. More than that, if we neglect our design to move, we are asking our brain to deteriorate.

In her book, *The Well Balanced Child*, Sally Goddard Blythe points out that one of the first signs of brain deterioration is when balance begins to deteriorate.[26] Why would brain deterioration and balance deterioration be linked together like this? Because your vestibular system keeps your brain healthy. If we don't use it, we lose it.

Fortunately for us, the "use it or lose it" principle is also the "use it to build it" principle. That road runs both ways! If we want a healthy vestibular system, we have to engage in using it; all we have to do is begin to live in our design.

The Brilliance of Big Heavy Heads

Have you ever considered the design of the human body? It's actually awe-inspiring. Consider that of all the mammals in the world, humans are born fairly defenseless and ill-proportioned. We come into the world extremely weak and have an overly large, watermelon-sized head attached to a tiny body. This is brilliant!

As a child, you built a healthy vestibular system, an amazing brain, and a resilient body by waging war against gravity. The head righting reflex made your body yearn to pick up and hold your humongous-sized head level with the horizon. You mastered this, and it was quite a miraculous feat of strength. Why? Because your head was insanely large compared to the rest of your tiny body. An infant's head weighs about 33% as much as its entire body weighs, and it is about 25% as big as its entire body. Yet, against the odds of physics and against the pull of gravity, you learned how to move your tiny body under your watermelon-sized head.

Think of it. Your head weighed 33% as much as your helpless little body, and you learned how to pick it up and hold it effortlessly on the horizon.

Let's have some fun and explore this with simple math. What if your head weighed 33% as much as your body today? Imagine if you only weighed 100 pounds. Your head would weigh 33 pounds! Can you imagine navigating through this life with a 33-pound head? You would be ridiculously strong if your head weighed that much. Do you see the brilliance in the design?

As a baby, you persistently and consistently labored to hold your head level with the horizon. You eventually mastered this and learned how to move your body underneath your head. This is how you tied your body, your X, together. This is how you developed ridiculous strength once upon a time.

Remember, your vestibular system is connected to every muscle in your body, especially the core musculature of the abdominals and back. It is these muscles that first work together to move the head.[27] When a child picks up his gargantuan-sized head while lying on the floor, he is developing his core, the center of his X, and he is becoming amazingly strong.

I once watched a friend's baby hold his head up for over 5 minutes while lying on the floor. He was on his belly, and the only thing touching the floor was his belly! His head was held high to see the world, and his arms and legs were intermittently held off the ground. He was doing a right-side-up "back bridge" while pivoting around in circles on his belly.

This fascinated me, so I tried it. I managed to make it through a brutal 5 minutes; it wasn't easy. I was shaking with muscular trimmers after the first minute. For the next two days, my backside was extremely sore. Even walking hurt. I only held that right-side-up back bridge for 5 minutes. The baby did it for 5 minutes at a time throughout the entire day. There are trade-offs to be sure between a child's body and an adult's body. My limbs were much longer than the baby's, but his head was relatively larger and heavier than mine. Either way, the baby was stronger and more well-conditioned for tummy time than I was.

This is because babies develop amazing strength. They develop this strength for their future selves. Adults should also have amazing strength because our younger selves set us up for it. In reality, we do have amazing strength tucked away in our design. We just may not have access to our strength because we are not living and moving in our design.

Today, adults don't really move their heads too often, and this could be the unraveling thread. If every muscle in the body is connected to the vestibular system, and movement of the head affects every muscle in the body, then not moving the head also affects every muscle in the body in a negative way. Not moving the head is like not stimulating all the muscles of the body. When muscles are not stimulated, they atrophy. When neural connections are unused, they get pruned or fade away. This is how weakness happens; it appears in the absence of strength.

The Power of Head Nods

For the last few decades, there has been a growing trend in the exercise world towards making the simple complicated—especially when it comes to the neck and spine. Ideas seem to be getting misapplied. Specifically, exercise rules and ideas are getting mis-applied in the area of natural human movement. In fact, some of the recommendations do not take into account how the body is actually designed to move, ignoring the integration of the body's reflexes and the body's design to follow the head.

In the fitness industry, it has become popular to encourage "packing the neck" or holding a "neutral spine" when performing exercises like squats and deadlifts. Packing the neck is a combination of cervical retrusion and capital flexion. So, two things are happening simultaneously—flexion and extension. Packing the neck or trying to hold a neutral spine is relatively safe, but it is not how the human body is designed to move. I say "relatively safe" because packing the neck can inhibit your strength and prevent you from moving in your design.

You've heard this before, but where the head goes, the body will follow. This is true. Regarding movement, we are designed so that the head leads the body. This means that when the head and neck move into extension, it facilitates extension in the body; the body wants to open up. When the head and neck move into flexion, it facilitates flexion in the body; the body wants to fold up. The same is true for rotation. Where the eyes and head lead, the body is wired to follow.

This is why keeping a packed neck or trying to hold a neutral spine could rob a person of their full strength expression. If we initiate movement with our head, our body is wired to follow that movement. Suppose we hold our eyes and our head still in a particular posture. In that case, we are dampening our body's reflexive wiring and strength, thus inhibiting our full strength expression potential. I'll even go as far as to say that if we are packing the neck and trying to hold flexion and extension simultaneously, we are essentially playing a game of tug-o-war inside of our nervous system. This mixed signal will not allow full expression of strength and power.

But for the sake of keeping friends in the exercise and fitness world, if you believe you should pack your neck and keep your spine in a neutral position while lifting weights, please do so. If it makes you feel safe, that feeling of safety helps your brain feel safe, and that's important when you're under heavy loads. But if you understand the design of your body to move, you can take that understanding into the weight room and apply it to your lifts. You can even test this with light to moderate loads in your lifts. Feel what a light to moderate deadlift feels like with your neck packed or with a neutral spine. Then, feel what a light to moderate deadlift feels like with your eyes and head held on the horizon. Whichever way feels the best to you or feels stronger, faster, and easier, do that!

Whatever route you take in the weight room or outside of the weight room, don't confuse exercise with natural human movement, and don't try to apply your exercise rules inside of natural movement. There is no need to pack the neck or hold a neutral spine when you are simply exploring your design to move. This means if you're crawling, it is okay and very good to hold your head and gaze up on the horizon.

For the purposes of Pressing RESET and helping you rediscover your original strength, I encourage you to move your head deliberately through full, pain-free ranges of motion. For simplicity's sake, I will call these motions head nods and head rotations.

Let's examine why head nods and head rotations are so powerful and important.

A quick Google search will tell you that the average person sits over 8 hours a day. Some estimates report that the average person in America sits for nearly 15 hours daily. It should go without saying, but if you were designed to move, sitting for 8 to 15 hours daily would be considered not living in your design. In fact, more and more, sitting is essentially like pouring yourself into a container known as a chair. For most of us, it's a full-on flexion position that is held and supported by the shape of the chair; it requires NO use of our postural muscles.

According to the SAID Principle (Specific Adaptation to Imposed Demand), the body adapts to what it repeatedly does. So when you're always sitting or filling your chair, your body gets stuck in flexion, and the muscles that support your posture are no longer needed to the degree they would be if you spent your time standing and moving.

Sitting shortens and tightens your flexors, lengthening and weakening your extending postural muscles. This is especially true if you are sitting and melting into the shape of your chair - you don't need back support; you need a back! When we sit like this, we are held by the chair or our facia. We are not being held by our musculature. Our core and postural muscles don't have to work at all when we sit like this; thus, they become weak and slow to respond. Remember, if we don't use it, we lose it.

But also remember, what we use, we build. Sitting in full flexion or a "fetus" position all day is *using* that position to fortify and develop that position.

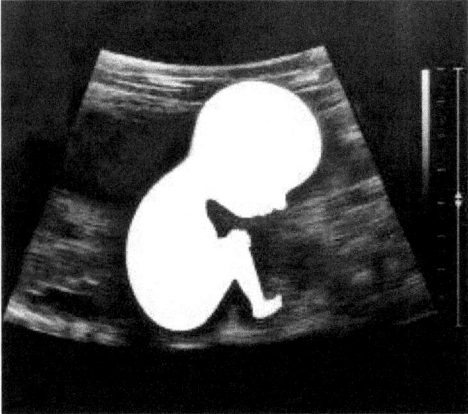

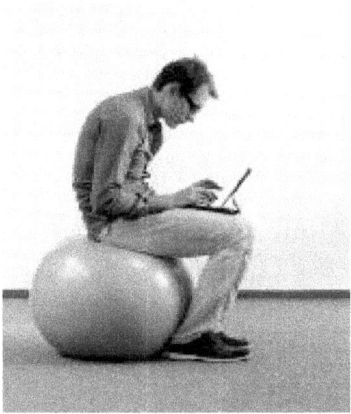

So when we stand, we end up resembling the shape of a question mark (?). We stand with a weird lower back posture and a rounded upper back, creating a forward head posture.

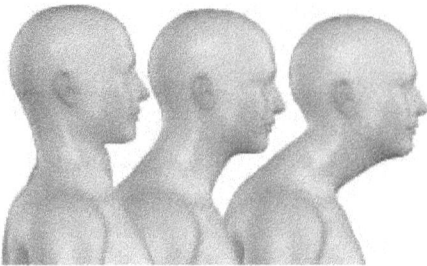

The further out the head is, the more it "weighs" through the leverage it creates. This places a large amount of stress on the spine and further comprises the body.

The path to restoration of posture - a true reflex—and the head control that determines it is found through exploring both flexion and extension. It may help to think of flexion as looking down and extension as looking up.

Suppose you ever watch a child developing, especially in the tummy-time months. In that case, you'll notice one thing: His head position is determined by his eye position. Wherever his gaze is, his head follows. If he looks up, his head follows, and his neck moves into extension. If he looks down, and his neck moves into flexion. If he looks left or right with his eyes, his head rotates to follow the eyes.

This is normal *and natural*. This natural motion strengthens his neck muscles, upper and lower back, and abs. In other words, when a baby is developing its head control, it is strengthening its core. For a baby, learning how to control his head is critical for his development of posture, balance, and coordination. In other words, head control is critical for the development and expression of his *strength*.

Again, this is a key concept to grasp: When you lose reflexive control of your head and neck, you lose your posture, your balance, and your coordination. The loss of coordination can be seen in everything from your reflexes to the visual tracking necessary to catch a ball. It can even be a symptom of a loss of mobility in the rest of your joints, like the thoracic spine, shoulders, hips, and ankles.

Do you see what's happening here? These losses in balance, posture, and coordination are typically seen as the consequences of aging. But these are not losses or deterioration due to a person's chronological age; these are losses and deterioration due to the neglect of movement.

If anything, not moving *is* aging.

This is one of the reasons we use head nods to begin building and regaining reflexive control of the head. Moving the head restores and builds the reflexive connections between the vestibular system and the postural and core musculature of the body.

Head nods are very simple to perform. The basic head nod starts on all fours—quadruped. (They can be performed in many other positions.) While on your hands and knees, simply look down and nod your chin to your chest, then look up with your eyes and lift your head up into extension as high as your body will allow. Don't force the movement; just explore the movement. Repeat this back and forth, up and down. *Make sure to keep your tongue on the roof of your mouth. This facilitates smooth neck movement.*

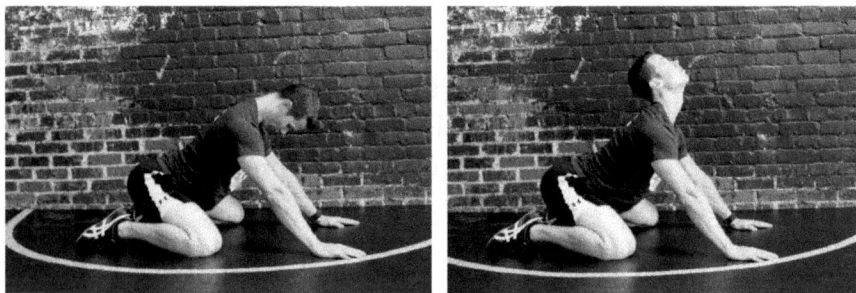

If you consistently engage in head nods, you'll find that they can unlock an immobile thoracic spine (a tight, stiff upper back), loosen up tight hips, and even help unlock frozen ankles. Gaining head control leads to body control.

Incidentally, as head control is reestablished, you'll find that your posture improves. Posture is a reflex, an expression of the health of your nervous system. It is not a position that you cognitively hold, nor can it be. Posture happens when your stabilizing muscles hold your body so that your moving muscles can efficiently move your body.

True posture is not a cognitively held position because cognitive muscles are moving muscles, not stabilizing muscles. Moving muscles tire fast when trying to be used as stabilizing postural muscles. No matter how much willpower you have, you cannot cognitively hold yourself in such a way that "good," reflexive posture just takes root and happens. You'll eventually tire out or forget to hold yourself in that desired position, and your "good" posture will evaporate in an instant.

Anyway, every single muscle in your body is tied to the movements of your head. Head and neck nods help restore these connections along with your natural movement reflexes so that you don't have to be concerned about your head and neck position or posture. This is because head nods help your body to do what it was reflexively designed to do without you having to think about it.

What Exactly Do Head & Neck Nods Do?

Head nods are an extremely powerful RESET, but why? And how do they work?

According to OS Master Instructor Dr. Mike Musselman, DC, the Head Nods are incredibly powerful from a neuro-mechanical perspective because:

- The specialized sensory cells of the upper cervical spine that communicate with your brain have a direct connection with the vestibular nuclei. This means they are not filtered by other parts of the brain because this is extremely important information for the brain to have. When the head moves only 0.4°, the brain detects this movement!
- The vestibular nuclei are responsible for maintaining your upright posture. Activation of these nuclei helps strengthen your postural patterns.

- Due to the high number of these specialized sensory cells in the upper cervical spine, head movement is fantastic for brain nourishment.
- Upper cervical spine sensory input has direct connections with the brain stem nuclei, which relay that information directly to the *nucleus tractus solitarious*, a part of the brain that helps regulate the immune system, the gastrointestinal system, the heart, and the lungs. Scientific evidence shows that input from the upper cervical spine is necessary to properly regulate these critically important body systems.

In layman's terms, head nods not only restore posture but can also help your body's major systems (immune, digestive, cardiovascular, and respiratory systems) function better and optimally.

Therefore, regaining head control by routinely performing head & neck nods is critically important for your overall health and well-being. And, if you were paying attention to what was said above, head nods may even help you turn back the clock on the traditional signs of aging by restoring your balance, posture, and coordination.

Plus, they help you feel amazing!

Keep Holding Your Tongue

Remember, tongue position matters. Placing your tongue in the "home" position, on the roof of your mouth behind your front teeth, is the reset within the RESETS.

In fact, placing the tongue on the roof of the mouth stimulates the tongue ligaments, which are connected to the vestibular system.[28] It also frees up the neck's range of motion, engaging the hyoid muscle group on the front of the neck, which reduces shear forces in the cervical vertebrae. This is important, as moving the head and neck has the fastest, most direct impact on the vestibular system. Suppose the vestibular system is activated and stimulated regularly by moving the neck through its full range of motion. In that case, the whole body is improved, resulting in a sharper vestibular system, a more efficient brain, and a better-moving, more connected, stronger body. This cannot fully happen without the tongue resting on the roof of the mouth.

Not only that, but people who rest their tongue on the bottom of their mouth tend to be mouth breathers, AND they also tend to have a forward head carriage. This means they are not breathing in their design, AND their head is not positioned above their shoulders as it should be. The more forward the head is held, the more the head "weighs" and strains the cervical spine. If the head is tilted 15°, it places about 27 pounds of force on the spine. If the head is tilted 30°, it places 40 pounds of force on the spine.[29]

Remember, the adult head is only supposed to weigh about 10 pounds! Breathing through the mouth and having a forward head carriage sends the message "I am not safe" to the brain and places extra strain on the body's structure. This is a stressor that keeps the body from expressing its full strength and health potential.

The point is to keep your tongue where it belongs. This encourages diaphragmatic breathing, helps restore your posture, and allows your neck to move freely, as it should. This is foundational to your overall health and well-being.

Say "Yes" to Head Nods (get it?):

- Start on your hands and knees, like you're about to crawl (quadruped).
- Keep your mouth closed.
- Place (rest) your tongue on the roof of your mouth. Again, if you're not sure exactly where this position is or

how it should feel, just swallow, and your tongue will go there automatically.

- Look down at your chest and nod your chin to your chest.
- Look up at the ceiling and raise your head as high as your neck will allow you to move.
- Nod your head up and down. Lead with your eyes!
- DO NOT MOVE INTO PAIN OR DIZZINESS, but move where you can move.
- Practice diaphragmatic breathing while performing your head nods. Do not hold your breath.
- Head Nods can be done in any position: lying on your back or belly, sitting, standing, on all fours, etc.

For more information, here is a playlist for head control movements:

https://youtube.com/playlist?list=PL9v3pv_KGM7vP6VfI7-2WnEYl_sGLQehn&si=4OWYVmHPVMx7Vz3c

Keep Your Head Up

"*While pregnant with my second child, I had debilitating back, hip, and leg pain. This continued for over 3 years. The pain also traveled into my neck, causing numbness and issues in my hands, feet, arms, legs, and face. I also developed walking issues. One or both of my legs would give out (think drunk stumbling girl here) up to 100 times a day. My neck pain was so intense it was hard to lift my head off my pillow or look right and left.*

I was sent to see 11 different doctors who told me I have/could have Multiple Sclerosis, Fibromyalgia, Ankylosing Spondylitis, Piriformis Syndrome, bulging discs, and/or sciatica. I was also told exercising more would fix these issues. I was already lifting kettlebells 3 times a week, walking, and participating in yoga or Pilates on other days. I was confused, embarrassed, and hurting. After receiving treatment plans that contained only pain pills and muscle relaxers, I was fed up.

Last February, I saw your video online speaking about relieving migraines by performing neck nods. I immediately tried them and have not looked back at the past once. I have looked up, down, and sideways. I remedied myself with the daily five RESETS religiously and tried a chiropractor for the first time. I wanted a natural cure for this awful pain that had gone on for so long. I wanted to be off these medications. I wanted to play with my sweet babies without pain for the first time.

Last June was my 9th and last chiropractic appointment as we were moving, and I did not know of a chiropractor in our new town. I have not been back to a chiropractor since, but I continue to practice OS daily and train with my kettlebells at least 3 times a week.

Last July, I received my MRI results showing all discs that had been bulging were totally normal and back in place! The pain became less and less, and now, coming a year later, I am totally pain-free! I had forgotten what it was like not to hurt! Sitting, standing, driving, holding my children does not hurt! My walking has also improved. My legs have only given out 7 times in the last four months. I am off all pain medications and muscle relaxers. In short, I have experienced a miracle!

I know God does not make mistakes and led me to OS for a reason. I want to tell the world what I have experienced! If I can help one person learn how to ease pain through all of this it will have been worth the years of hurting.

I wish doctors knew how to recommend such a movement system, especially for mommies. I tell everyone I know about OS, and they all want to learn about it. Every time I show someone the RESETS, they laugh. I believe it is the God-given movement patterns and childlike quality that cause this. As laughter is the best medicine, I will continue to show everyone OS and will practice it for life.

Thank you for giving me this gift. Please let me know how to share it with others. Thank you for taking the time to read my story, and may God Bless you!"

Sincerely,
Amber Harrison, mom
Georgia

"P.S. I'm sorry if this is too wordy and long; I tried to condense it. THREE years is a long time, and doctors told me so many different things that I wasn't sure what to put in here. Thank you again for listening and for your time :)"

Know Your Roll

Before my first son, Luke, could crawl, I often placed him on the floor in the middle of the room, thinking it was a safe place for him. He would play, and I would do some work on the computer. But that all changed when Luke discovered how to roll. One time, *the last time*, I placed Luke on the floor and turned around to check my email and pay some bills on the computer. I turned around to check on him, but he wasn't there. He had rolled to the other side of the room. It was an impressive distance. Apparently, something over there had caught his attention. From that day on, my days of working on the computer while Luke had tummy time were over.

As children, rolling is how we learn to get to the objects that beg for our curiosity. Rolling is the true foundation of our gait pattern, as it is our first method of locomotion. When a child learns how to roll, he further ties his X together. Building on top of the strength that breathing and gaining head control establish, rolling is where the child starts connecting the opposite shoulder to the opposite hip, anteriorly and posteriorly (it connects the front side of your X and the back side of your X). Rolling adds another layer of strength to the child's center.

When a child learns to roll, he develops rotational strength and stability. This strength prepares his body for the rotational forces that walking and running will produce. This rotational stability also allows the child's trunk to remain stable under asymmetrical and contralateral loads, a critical component of spinal health. This rotational strength is also reflexive, allowing the child to develop balance and control over his movements.

Remembering how to roll around on the floor is key to restoring the strength we were designed to have. Everything rolling does for the developing child still holds true for the "redeveloping" adult. It is also worth mentioning that rolling is crucial to keeping your spine young and healthy. In case you have forgotten or in case you didn't know, your spine was made to rotate, and rotation nourishes the spine.

Adults should be able to roll around on the floor easily, just like children can. However, this is not always the case, as we have often witnessed during the Original Strength Screen and Assessment (OSSA). In the OSSA, rolling can quickly reveal how well connected a person's body is—whether or not their shoulders are connected to their hips and whether or not they have rotational strength and stability, among other things.

Again, we should all be able to roll around on the floor easily, but not everyone can. For many adults, rolling takes a lot of strain and effort. However, the ease of rolling can be restored by investing a little time on the floor exploring how to roll. Effortless rolling builds a healthy nervous system, resulting in tremendous strength and health! A fluid X is a strong X.

Rolling Your Brain Together

Rolling doesn't just tie the X together on the outside. It also builds a very healthy brain. When you roll, you are greatly activating your vestibular system and further developing head control. You are also stimulating your skin, the largest sensory organ you possess. Your skin receives and transmits all kinds of information about you and your environment. It is always a feeling for information. It detects how cold you are, how humid it is, what kind of surface you are touching, how hard something is touching you, etc.... Some even refer to the skin as the "outer brain" because it receives so much information. In fact, the skin contains 640,000 sensory receptors that are connected to the spinal cord by over 500,000 neural pathways![30] It is like a great big nerve in and of itself.

Rolling nourishes your brain through information. Your brain craves information about you and your surroundings. With this information, the brain is asking that same question, "Am I safe?" Not receiving the information the brain is expecting and craving, or not receiving any information because the body is sedentary, is the same as sending incomplete or missing information. Missing information is a safety issue. In a sense, it starves the brain and causes the brain to feel unsafe, thus putting the body in the sympathetic fight or flight state.

In fact, scientists have learned that children who don't receive loving touch (skin stimulation and attention) from a caregiver actually suffer from the same effects as undernourishment, including retarded bone growth, poor muscular coordination, immunological weakness, and general apathy.[31] In case you are wondering, a "loving touch" can be someone rocking a child to sleep, calming them by rubbing their back, or simply playing with them. Loving touch provides tactile information to the brain as well as positional information about the child's body.

Like loving touch, rolling provides the brain with this same nourishing information. Remember, your vestibular system receives all sensory information from the body and sends this information to the brain. All the stimulation and activation that rolling generates feeds your brain with "safe" nourishment. Every time you roll, you give your brain rich information that either creates new neural connections (nerve pathways in your brain) or cements the neural connections you already have. The more information you generate through your natural human movements, like rolling, the "safer" your brain determines it is. And, the more neural connections you have, and the more ingrained they become, the more efficient your brain becomes. This allows for quicker thought, stable emotions, and an optimal expression of functional movement patterns.

It's wild to think, but rolling can keep your brain healthy, allowing you to become a better thinker and a better mover. Rolling doesn't just help make you healthier and stronger; it helps to make you whole. But then, so does loving touch.

How Do You Roll?

Rolling is simply the act of lying on the floor and transitioning from your belly to your back and from your back to your belly. There are more ways to roll than there are letters in the alphabet. In this book, we will discuss the Segmental Roll presented in Gray Cook's book, *Movement*. This roll works wonders in restoring reflexive strength and cleaning up movement patterns.

Segmental Rolling:[32]

- Back to Belly Rolling—Upper Body:
  - Lie on your back with your legs straight and your arms straight overhead.
  - **Using your head**, neck, and right arm, reach diagonally across your body, over your left hip, as far as you can, and roll to your belly.
  - **Try not to use your legs! Keep them relaxed.**

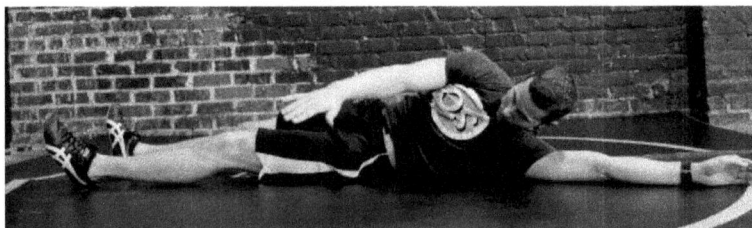

- Belly to Back Rolling—Upper Body:
  - Lie on your belly with your legs straight and your arms straight overhead.

o **Use your head**, neck, and right arm to reach back across your body and roll to your back. Try to watch your hand touch the floor behind you.

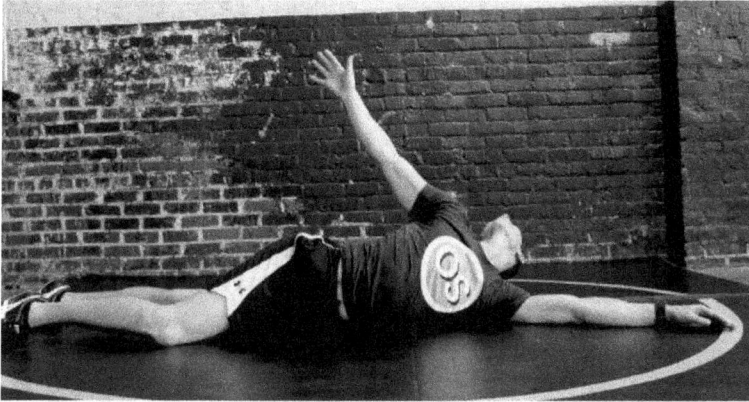

- Back to Belly Rolling—Lower Body:
  o Lie on your back with your legs straight and your arms straight overhead.
  o Using your right leg, reach up and across your body and roll to your belly. Imagine you are reaching for an object with your foot all the way across the room.
  o **Try not to use your arms. Keep them relaxed.**
  o Can you do this with equal movement and effort with both legs?

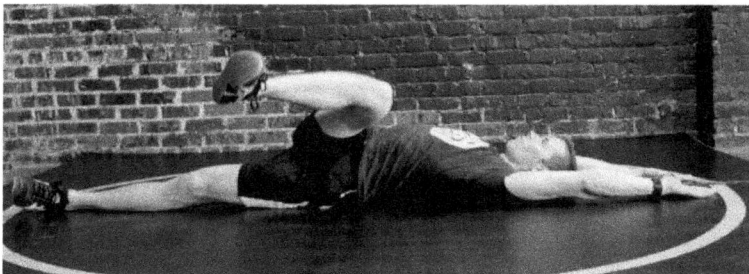

- Belly to Back Rolling—Lower Body:
  o Lie on your belly with your legs straight and your arms straight overhead.
  o Use your right leg to reach back across your body and roll to your back. It may help to imagine that you are reaching for an object with your foot all the way across the room.
  o Can you do this with equal movement and effort with both legs?

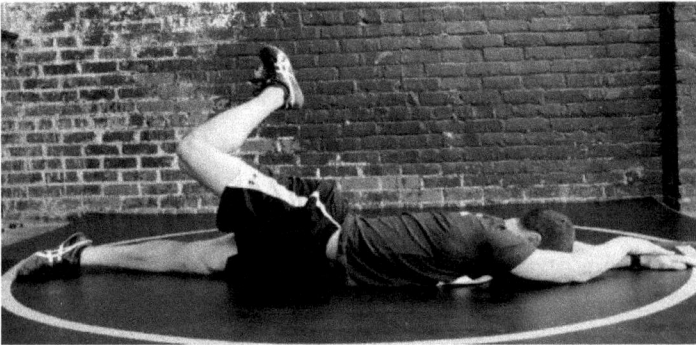

Even though babies don't roll as deliberately as I do in the pictures, they do roll segmentally. They are incredibly fluid and roll "piece by piece," segment by segment, almost like an ocean wave. You should be able to roll this way, too.

The Segmental Roll is a great roll to explore when it comes to rolling. I like to teach my clients to roll this way because it can expose movement issues and unlock movement issues at the same time. At the Original Strength Institute, I've witnessed rolling "fix" or cleanup an entire Functional Movement Screen Score[33] instantly at the speed of my clients' nervous systems. This makes sense because rolling is programmed deep inside our original operating system. It is one of the first ways we start to learn and develop our movement patterns as infants. Rolling is also a great way to relearn and rebuild our movement patterns again as adults.

Pressing RESET: Original Strength Forever

In the Segmental Roll, eight rolling patterns are involved. The rolls go from belly to back, back to belly, left to right, right to left, right arm, left arm, right leg, and left leg. Ideally, all eight of those patterns should be of equal ease; they should all be fluid and effortless. However, some of these patterns may be difficult for some people. Some of these patterns may not even be currently possible for other people—they can't perform the Segmental Roll yet.

Oftentimes, simply spending time on the floor and exploring the Segmental Roll can restore these patterns. In other words, rolling makes *rolling* better. At other times, the Segmental Roll may need to be broken down into smaller, less complicated rolls that we call regressions. These regressions are explored in detail in the Pressing RESET training courses.

Once Segmental Rolling can be performed with ease, other forms of rolling can be introduced. The following rolls are more advanced rolls. These are just examples of different ways to roll. They need not be performed if Pressing RESET on the body is all that is desired. However, these rolls are fun and a great way to play and explore one's strength and control. Spending time exploring challenging rolls will sharpen and improve the body's ability to move.

The Head Roll:

- While resting on your forearms and belly, use only your head and neck and roll over to your back. You should end up on your back with your legs straight and your arms resting over your chest.

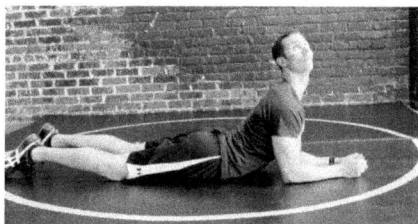

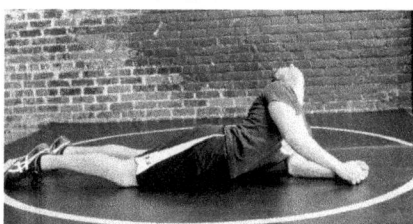

- While lying on your back, use only your eyes, head, and neck and roll to your belly.
- You should aim to "land" propped up on your forearms.

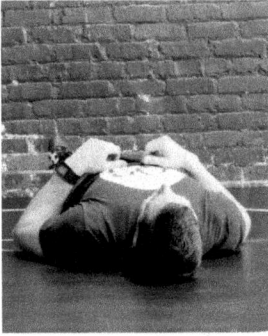

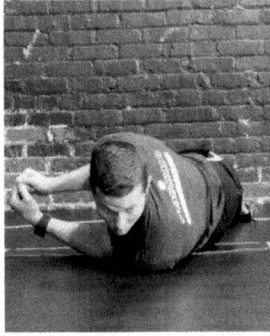

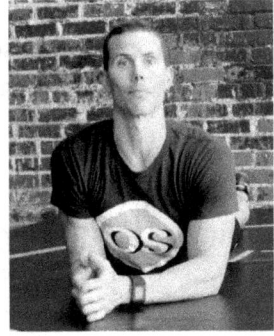

- Practice rolling in both directions.
- This is an upper body segmental roll without the use of the arms.

The Elevated Roll:

- Assume the push-up plank position on your hands and feet.
- Use your right leg to reach back across your body and roll until your right foot rests on the ground.
- As you reach and roll with your right leg, your right hand will eventually be pulled along until it leaves the ground.
- When your right foot makes contact with the ground, your right arm will end up pointing up at the sky.
- Push both feet into the ground and reach for the sky with your pelvis. (Perform a hip bridge.)
- When you are ready to return, REACH across your body with your right hand and drive it down towards the ground beside your left hand. This will pull your lower body back over to the starting push-up plank position.

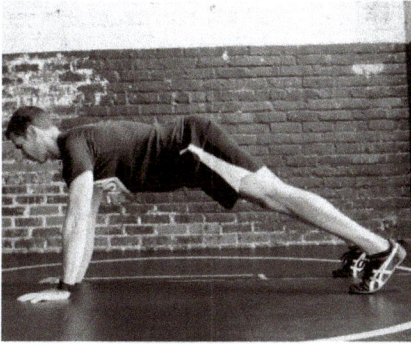

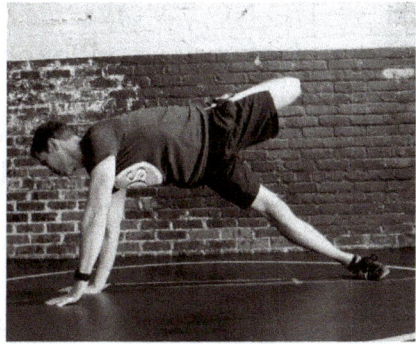

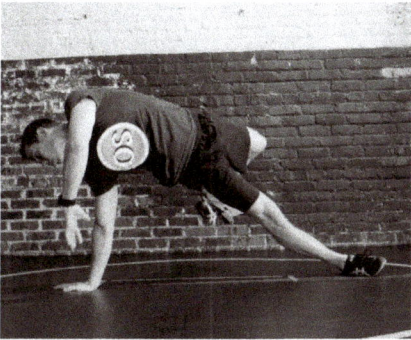

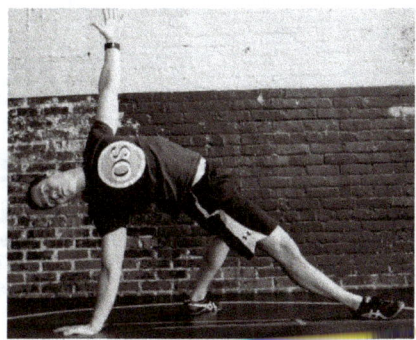

The elevated roll feels fantastic! It can make a great "movement snack" to throw into your day every now and then. It also looks really cool at parties!

Rolling Tips

- Remember, the body is designed to follow the head, and the head is designed to follow the eyes! When rolling from the upper body, lead with your eyes and use your head.
- Keep your mouth closed.
- Place (rest) your tongue on the roof of your mouth.
- To roll fluidly and segmentally, you have to be able to "let go" and relax your body. This may be next to impossible if you haven't mastered diaphragmatic breathing yet.

- DO NOT MOVE INTO PAIN. You can roll to the edge of it but don't roll into it.
- It is okay to look like an accident. When you first begin to roll, it may not look so fluid. This is okay. Keep rolling. With time and effort, fluidity will come.

To see more rolling variations, here is a rolling playlist:

https://youtube.com/playlist?list=PL9v3pv_KGM7tMEavu
GEErSMOrhCRJv38N&si=vWbWr63tT8W7V3dL

The Impact of Rolling

"I've said it, and I'll say it again, I found rolling long ago, actually studying psychology and neurology. I was lucky enough to realize the value of the physical and 'life impact' and through digging and stumbling onto Original Strength very early on. Nothing I have found has had as big of an impact on correcting my client's movement, living life, and just flat-out being badasses."

—Matt Woodard, A.K.A. Kal-El
Florida

Welcome to the Rock

Once a child learns how to roll on purpose, they start building serious strength. Eventually, they learn how to press themselves up and away from the floor, where they learn to move from their hands and knees. A child develops a new layer of strength and coordination from this new position. Just holding this position builds strength in the child, especially with that large head trying to weigh it down. Remember that the child is programmed to move and is simply answering the call of the wild. And that call is loud and strong.

The child doesn't just want to hold this position; it wants to move from it. It wants to go from where it is now to where its curiosity is calling it. But in the beginning, when a child gets strong enough to get on its hands and knees, it doesn't quite have the strength or coordination to crawl yet. Instead, it has an internal movement pattern designed to build the strength and coordination needed for crawling: rocking.

Rocking back and forth is the movement pattern a child uses to build the structural integrity and coordination needed to get all four limbs working together to get from "here to there." It is cool to witness a child doing this. It almost looks as if they are trying to build enough momentum to get their body to crawl as if they are trying to overcome the inertia of being motionless. Yet, at the same time, it looks so joyful. Their faces are typically beaming when they rock back and forth.

Maybe children are joyful when they rock because they somehow know how amazing rocking is as a movement pattern. There is so much happening in the child's body when it rocks back and forth. Rocking is a complete integration movement; it integrates all parts of the body with the soul.

But let's start with what rocking does in the body. When a child begins rocking, he is basically providing his brain with all the information needed to learn that the body is one whole fluid being; it is not made of several parts and pieces. Rocking is where all the body's major joints learn how to move and dance together. The joints of the feet, the ankles, the knees, the hips, the pelvis, the spine, the shoulders, and the wrist all move together in unison and become integrated into the brain. Rocking teaches the brain where all the moving parts are and how to coordinate all those moving parts together.

Rocking also reflexively integrates the body's muscles, especially those that surround all those dancing joints. Rocking back and forth teaches the child's "stabilizers" (like the rotator cuffs of the shoulder) how to hold and stabilize the joints. It teaches the child's "movers" (like the deltoids of the shoulder) how to move the joints. In other words, when a child rocks back and forth on his hands and knees, he is building reflexive stability *and* mobility throughout his entire body.

But remember, stability *is* mobility *is* control *is* strength. These are all expressions of movement and these expressions are all developed together when we move through our design.

Rocking does two other things for us physically that are also quite amazing.

Rocking teaches our opposing limbs how to mirror one another. It primes us for our contralateral gait pattern by teaching our opposite shoulders how to dance with our opposite hips. This leads us down the path to being able to crawl, walk, skip, and run beautifully. But it also leads us down the path to better brain health and development. The mirroring motion of our opposing limbs develops and integrates both hemispheres of our brain, improving our brain's ability to function and communicate with our body.

Rocking also sets our spine's curves and helps us reflexively establish optimal posture. The quadruped position, being on the hands and knees, is where the cervical curve (the neck curve) and the lumbar curve (the lower back curve) become established. This position sets the shape of our spine and teaches our core muscles how to reflexively respond to maintain optimal posture. Remember, posture is reflexive but also dynamic. It is not a held, static position. It is expression.

True posture cannot be cognitively held with muscular effort. It just *is*. And what it *is* is a result of the information we feed our brain through movement. If you want to see the state of health in a person's nervous system, look at their postural expressions. How do they hold themselves? How do they move? This will also give you insight into the state of their soul. How do they feel? What are their emotions expressing to you? How they hold themselves and how they move can tell you more about their current state than words ever need to say.

There is no separation in us. Our emotions affect how we move, and our movements affect how we emote.

This is the other "non-physical" thing that rocking does. It soothes our souls. This movement helps to integrate the entire body and soul as one.

Soothe Your Soul

If you've been fortunate enough to be a parent, you have undoubtedly rocked your child to soothe and comfort them. You intuitively knew how to do this, but you also *had* to do it because love spurred you to do it. Somewhere inside all of us, we know that rocking soothes the soul. Perhaps it is because rocking is rhythmic, perhaps it's because rocking activates the vestibular system in a similar way that an unborn baby experiences the walking motion of its mother, or perhaps our brains just love steady, predictable patterns. Whatever the reason, rocking tethers our minds and emotions to our movement.

Movement does build our brains by creating neural pathways. But movement also helps to build our minds and regulate our emotions. A mind that doesn't receive movement can become restless and agitated, which often leads to uncontrollable emotions. You already know this to be true.

What do agitated children who are having trouble with their emotions do? What does an irate adult who is perhaps ready to fight do? They rock, or sway, or pace. It is all the same: They move back and forth to soothe and calm their emotions. They rock to "RESET" their emotions. As we learned earlier, the brain craves information. Rocking is a movement that floods the brain with a great deal of "safe" information.

It stimulates the vestibular system and nourishes the brain and body, much like good food nourishes the brain and body. Movement keeps the nerves from "unraveling" and the emotions from "unhinging." The problem is that we get corralled into living sedentary lives in our modern world. Is it any wonder that many Americans are frazzled and stressed out? We live in a world that encourages not moving.

If a movement like rocking back and forth can help reduce and relieve stress, then the opposite is also true. Not moving can perpetuate stress and exasperate the mind. How easy is it to think and make rational decisions when you are upset? How easy is it to be kind and present your true self to others when you are anxious or angry? Our emotions are tethered to our movements. We can move ourselves to peace and calm, to patience and kindness, by Pressing RESET with movements like rocking.

By the way, many parents instinctively hum or sing soft lullabies to their crying babies as they rock them. Humming stimulates the vestibular system and helps calm the emotions.[34] A humming, rocking parent is not only calming the upset child; they are also soothing their own nerves.

The next time you get upset, try humming while you rock. You may find that it works wonders to settle you and soothe your soul.

Rock On

Rocking is a powerful RESET. I've seen it restore the mobility of feet, ankles, knees, hips, shoulders, and wrists. It can relieve lower back pain and discomfort, enhance posture, and correct many other movement issues. My good friend and world-famous strength and conditioning coach and author, Dan John, credits rocking for rehabbing his hips after having undergone hip replacement surgeries. Since his surgeries, Dan has competed in the Highland Games and is still enjoying and competing in Olympic Weightlifting meets, which is his passion. Rocking reintegrated Dan's new hips into his body and reconnected his X, allowing him to engage in the joys of his life. Dan even told me rocking calms and relaxes him when he's stressed. If you know Dan, you know he is full throttle with high energy and passion. You also know he doesn't waste time on movements or ideas that don't work. Rocking works so well that Dan shares it with all his students, friends, and clients. It's wild how powerful this movement is when you consider how simple it is to perform.

Rocking is performed by getting down on your hands and knees, keeping a "proud" chest, and holding your eyes and head up on the horizon. From this position, simply push your butt back towards your feet. Then, rock forward, placing your weight back over your hands.

Back and forth, forth and back...

In the beginning, take it nice and slow. As you get comfortable with it, you can play with the speed you rock. As your hips loosen up, you can also play with the width in which you place your knees by moving them closer together or farther apart. You can also rock using different foot positions. There is no "one way" to rock. Playing and exploring the different rocking positions and motions can be very relaxing and therapeutic.

While there is no one way to rock, be sure to hold your head up when rocking, at least in the beginning and for the majority of the time. When a child rocks back and forth, the righting reflex encourages his head to be held up on the horizon. Your head should remember where the horizon is, too. Remember, rocking is where we restore and reset our posture.

But also remember that the body is designed to follow the head; you are reflexively wired together by the movements and positions of your head. In fact, you can see how this works for yourself. From the bottom rocking position, while you are sitting back over your calves, perform some Head Nods. You will feel your whole back musculature respond and "turn on" as your head is lifted up. If you set your head level with the horizon and then try to look over your shoulders to see your "back pockets," you will feel your lats (big "muscle wings" on your back). The muscles around your scapula pull your shoulder blades down towards your butt. Head motion and position initiate the reflexive responses and actions of your postural and core muscles.

Rocking also helps make our center stronger by engaging our pelvic muscles, causing them to reflexively fire as we rock back and forth. You may notice this as you push your butt back towards your calves, especially if you increase the speed at which your rock. If you focus on what you feel, you will likely notice your perineum area reflexively respond as you bounce back from the bottom of the rocking position. A reflexively strong pelvic floor is essential for overall strength and health. This is just another reason why rocking is so powerful.

Remember, as we grow and move through the developmental sequence, we add strength to our center layer by layer. Our original strength starts from the center out. It is built between a properly functioning diaphragm and a properly functioning pelvic floor. The diaphragm and the pelvic floor form the inner core; they make the center of the X solid and resilient.

Combining diaphragmatic breathing and rocking can be a powerful combination of RESETS to reestablish our strong and resilient centers. This is especially true for women trying to restore their bodies after childbirth. But, men, this is also especially true for you if you are trying to restore your resiliency after a lifetime of movement neglect or after experiencing physical and emotional trauma. You were made to heal. Rocking and breathing are movements that help you heal…

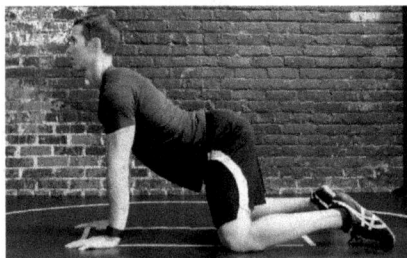

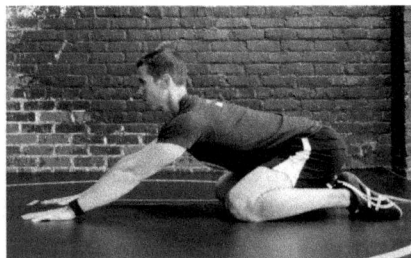

How to Perform Rocking:

- Start on your hands and knees as if you are about to crawl.
- In the beginning, place the tops of your feet on the ground (plantarflex your feet—laces down!)
- Keep a "proud" chest, like Superman.
- Hold your eyes and head up so that you can see the horizon.
- Push your butt back towards your feet.

Pressing RESET: Original Strength Forever

- Rock forward until your shoulders are over your hands.
- Move in and out, back and forth, slowly—at first.
- Play with different speeds as you get used to the motion.
- Play with different width positions for your knees.
- Don't forget to explore with Head Nods while holding the forward and back positions.
- Don't forget to explore nasal and diaphragmatic breathing while holding the forward and back positions.

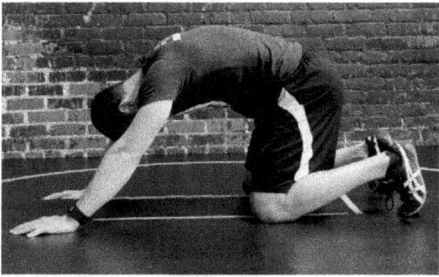

This is not what we want to do. Notice that the head is down, and the spine is round. Keep the head up and keep the spine "flat" by holding a proud chest.

You don't ever have to do this, but if you're curious and you want to use rocking as a way to "strength train", you can add a little extra resistance by performing elevated rocking on your hands and your feet. This places a much greater demand on your muscles, significantly increasing the tension needed to suspend your entire body weight in the air. You won't have to think about tightening your muscles; it happens automatically and reflexively.

Again, you don't have to do this, but it's an "easy" way to build strength while you integrate your whole body. Ok, it's not easy. It's actually quite brutal and uncomfortable. But if you ever get to the point where it becomes comfortable, you are strong and able on multiple levels! Elevated Rocking for time is a great way to build your "I can-ness," as in *I can do hard things.*

Rocking on Hands and Feet

- Start on your hands and feet.
- Keep a tall chest, like Superman.
- Hold your head up so you can see the horizon.
- Push your butt back towards your feet.
- Make sure you keep a proud chest!
- Make sure you breathe! Do not hold your breath.
- Move in and out, back and forth, slowly—at first.
- Play with different speeds as you get used to the motion.

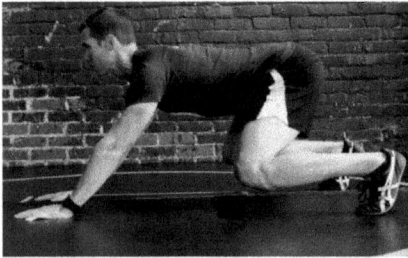

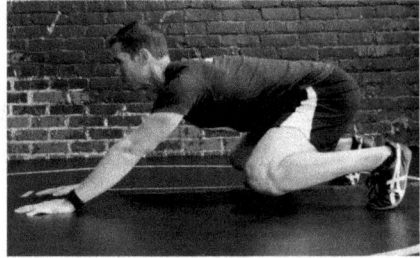

To see more rocking variations, here is a rocking playlist:

https://www.youtube.com/playlist?list=PL9v3pv_KGM7
vr3nz69wOff7vWsc4ix2jx

Movement is More Than a Physical Exercise

"I've completed my first month of Pressing RESET. Of twenty-four scheduled training days, I've trained twenty. I have done RESETS daily and sometimes several times daily.

I start each day by giving grace upon waking and then performing RESETS as I sit on the edge of my bed: breathing, head nods, rocking, and cross crawls. This is the best I have felt all year and the best I have felt spiritually, physically, and emotionally in a very long time.

I'm looking forward to my continued progress and journey of becoming the best person I can be and enjoying life to the fullest. Thank you for your help and guidance in this journey.

Be Blessed, Be Strong, Be Happy"

–Kirby Sams
Austin TX

Crawl Yourself Together

After a child relentlessly builds his strength through the consistent effort of pushing himself up and away from the floor and then rocking back and forth, he is ready to begin crawling. Crawling is the culmination of all the other developmental movements we've discussed. It results from diaphragmatic breathing, head control, the rotary stability and strength of rolling, and the whole-body integration of rocking. Crawling is the developmental movement that establishes THE foundation of the most graceful and capable creature ever to grace the planet—You.

Crawling ties *everything* about us together. It weaves us whole in nearly every imaginable way, even in many ways we never imagined. This may be hard to grasp, but as far as movements go, crawling is like the fountain of YOUth; it can restore you.

Pressing Reset With Cross-Lateral Movements

Crawling is a cross-lateral, or contra-lateral, movement that completes the foundation of the human gait pattern. (Remember, rolling is where we begin locomotion.) When we crawl or walk, our opposite limbs are supposed to move in coordination with each other; they mirror one another. This is the design of our X. This coordinated movement ties the brain, the body, and the brain *and* the body together.

How does crawling tie the brain together?

We touched on this briefly in the rocking section, but crawling combines two halves to make a whole. Your brain has two hemispheres: the right hemisphere, known as the gestalt side, and the left hemisphere, known as the logic side. Both hemispheres need to work well together for your body to be efficient at anything.[35] Performing cross-lateral movements and/or midline crossing movements increases the communication between the two hemispheres of your brain.[36] Midline crossing movements are movements that cross the middle line of your body. For example, taking your right hand and reaching for your left leg is a midline crossing movement.

Your neural plasticity, cross-lateral, and midline crossing movements cause the brain to make new neural connections between the two hemispheres. These movements literally tie the brain together by creating neural connections inside the brain, weaving both hemispheres of the brain together. Cross-lateral and midline crossing movements are crucial for learning and brain development. These movements are also vital to physical development. The more neural connections there are between the two hemispheres, the better the hemispheres can work together and communicate with the body.

In short, crawling helps to build and develop the brain. A healthy brain can more easily command, control, and protect the body, enabling the body to express its whole movement and strength potential. However, it also allows the mind to express its full potential in creativity and logic. It also enables the soul to regulate emotions and connect better with others. When we are better as human beings, we are better as neighbors, husbands, wives, sons, and daughters. Crawling weaves us whole in all areas of our lives.

> The pattern for crawling actually lives in the spinal cord, not the brain.

I know that sounds far-fetched, but let's look at it a little deeper. Crawling is not a recent evolutionary development in humans. It is the original gait template programmed into your great, great,

great grandfather and his great, great, great, grandfather. Since man began, crawling has been pre-programmed inside of man's operating system. The pattern for crawling actually lives in the spinal cord, not the brain. Isn't this wild?! If crawling builds the brain, doesn't it make sense that the crawling pattern lives in the spinal cord? The body is so wonderfully designed!

Anyway, we were all pre-programmed to crawl. However, not all of us do. For various reasons like germaphobic parents who are afraid to put their child on the floor, overly enthusiastic parents who rush their kids into walking, cultural norms, or any number of reasons, some children skip crawling or don't spend enough time crawling. There may be a consequence to moving through an entire crawling season, though. Research has shown that children who skip crawling are more likely to have learning disorders.[37] Their brains are not as "connected" as children who enjoy a more extended crawling season. They are also more likely to have movement and coordination issues as well because crawling sets the foundation for the gait pattern.

When you think about it, crawling is a highly complex movement pattern that simultaneously requires balance, stability, coordination, rhythm, strength, endurance, and breath. For the body to quickly and fluidly learn how to crawl, it must build a robust brain with intricate neural pathways capable of facilitating all of this orchestration. For this reason, it should be no surprise that research has also shown that crawling can help a person overcome learning disorders, if not be healed from them.

Maybe you were a person who didn't crawl. It doesn't matter. The program is still inside you, and you can still "run the program" and renew your nervous system, rebuild your brain, and restore your original strength. Even if you are 99 years young and haven't used that program for the last 88 years, it is still inside you waiting to be tapped into.

But again, crawling is not just great for the brain. It builds and myelinates your neural pathways, improving their ability to send and receive signals and making your reflexes more efficient and much faster. Again, crawling ties the X together; it builds and restores effortless strength and mobility. For example, through sensory nerves called mechanoreceptors in the hands and feet, crawling stimulates reflexive core musculature activation, which gets the shoulders and pelvis working together.[38]

At the risk of repeating myself, posture is a reflexive expression. In *The Well Balanced Child*, Sally Goddard Blythe points out, "Movement on all fours (like rocking and crawling) also helps to align the spine at the back of the neck with the sacral region in preparation for proper alignment in the upright posture."[39] Every step that is made when crawling on all four limbs stimulates these mechanoreceptors, activating the reflexive core musculature that connects the torso, aligns the spine, and establishes optimal upright posture.

You can see evidence of this reflexive response. Just watch a person's triceps contract when they crawl. Every step they take with their hands elicits a contraction in their triceps and all the other muscles in their body that you can't even see. Every step elicits a reflexive response throughout the entire body. Can you see the ridiculously gentle and reflexive strength training that is taking place here?

But wait! There is more!

Crawling enables us to express our full athleticism, even in ways we might not consider. It can improve our binocular vision, hand-eye coordination, and even binaural hearing (our perception of sound from two ears).[40] Crawling helps lay the foundation, on multiple levels, of who we become and how we express ourselves through movement.

Again, it weaves us into wholeness.

Crawling sounds quite miraculous. But how can it be? After all, we are only designed to crawl for such a short period of time relative to how long we live. We crawl to be able to walk. We are designed to be walkers, not crawlers.

This is all true. But it is also true that **we are not designed to sit around all day.**

And yet, that is what most of us do.

If you are following the line of thought from what I've presented about crawling, walking should be our default miraculous movement, the one that truly weaves us whole. But many of us could benefit from relearning how to crawl before walking. Crawling is *foundational* to walking. We can use crawling to reestablish healthy neural pathways and restore our reflexive foundation of strength. Once we do that, walking will be the most significant movement of human restoration and expression.

The reality is that most people do not walk in their design. Many walk and run without using their shoulders and arms properly. Some people walk around without even using their arms at all. The problem with this is that we have four limbs for gait; it takes four limbs to crawl, and it is supposed to take four limbs to walk. Instead of being walkers, many have become amblers and are not moving according to their design. As a result, they don't have the solid foundation they were made to have, and they cannot express their body's full strength and mobility potential. They are limited, and therefore, they are not as resilient and capable as they should be.

Crawling is the Great RESET. You can't really amble when you crawl. It requires the deliberate use of four limbs. The shoulders and hips have to work together in order to get from one place to another. Crawling RESETS the nervous system and returns walking to its intended cross-lateral gait pattern. When we walk as we were deigned, we are performing THE RESET we were all made to do, with every single step we take.

Learning to Crawl

If you decide to embark on crawling, and I hope you do, use patience and GOOD judgment. I will present some crawling options below, but honor your body and spend time crawling *where you are at the level your body can currently crawl.* In other words, be honest with yourself and start where you are. Start by crawling on your hands and knees if unsure where you are. I say this because many people want to jump right into the Spider-man crawl, but their bodies may not be ready for the demands of the Spider-man crawl. Believe it or not, some people are not ready for the demands of hands and knees crawling, either. You may be one of them, and that's ok, even good.

You need to start where you are, at the level, your body is ready to handle. The Spider-Man crawl is fantastic, and it can build the strength of your dreams, but so can crawling on your hands and knees—if you'll explore it with patience, honesty, and curiosity.

Hands and Knees Crawling

Hands and knees crawling is the gold standard of crawling. I only say that because when you think of crawling, you probably imagine it to be on your hands and knees, the way a baby would crawl. This is a seemingly simple movement, yet it is incredibly complex when considering the orchestration of motions and expressions the body must accomplish for crawling. Considering how the brain learns and develops from crawling is ridiculously brilliant and awe-inspiring.

The movement that requires balance, coordination, timing, rhythm, intent, strength, endurance, fluidity, control, and neural real estate in the brain is the movement that also builds, develops, and enhances these same things. The ease and mastery of crawling happen through the struggle of learning to crawl. Along this path, from struggle to mastery, the brain, nervous system, body, and soul develop and grow in resilience. I guess I'm saying that crawling on our hands and knees develops our "roots." It helps establish and nourish our neural roots so that our physical and mental structures can endure the storms of life.

Enough talk. The opposite limbs should move and work together when crawling on hands and knees. While two opposing limbs are being lifted and advanced, the other two opposing limbs support and suspend the body off the ground. Two limbs hold, and two limbs advance in a criss-cross fashion. The two moving limbs will advance and land almost simultaneously - every person has their own rhythm for this.

Some people are "Exact Jack" in the timing of their opposing limbs, and others have more of a *hand that moves slightly before their legs* move rhythm if traveling forward. Regardless, the moving opposing limbs should have a close rhythm that requires the body to stabilize on the other two opposing limbs. I know this seems like it doesn't need to be said, but the crawling pattern can be quite a bit "rusty" in some people, and they may have trouble coordinating this fluid, criss-cross motion.

Also, while crawling, hold your eyes and head up on the horizon to see the world. This further enhances the postural benefits of being on all fours. Do not try to hold your head level with your spine, or do not try to keep a neutral spine unless you are purposely looking for something on the ground. Your head may feel very heavy at first, but your neck will get stronger, especially if you challenge it by trying to hold your head up. If you must drop your head, just take a break and allow your neck to recover.

As best as you can, when you practice crawling, practice holding your eyes and head up.

Since we are practicing, when you practice crawling, also practice breathing through your nose with your tongue on the roof of your mouth. This is the best way to gently develop the strength of your diaphragm and cardiovascular system. If your mouth pops open to breathe, that is your body telling you that you've currently exceeded your ability to maintain nasal breathing, and it needs to REST. So rest.

Yes, you could "easily" continue to crawl while breathing through your mouth, but that only reinforces a breathing pattern you do not want. We don't want to teach and enable our bodies to do what we don't want. We want to return to our design. This means we want our body to remember how to perform work while nasal breathing efficiently. We want each breath to tell the brain we are safe even when training and practicing our movements.

Practice your desired qualities, and ask your body for what you want by challenging its capabilities and honoring its design. However, whatever you train, think, or do is what you are asking your body for. Therefore, train the motions and qualities you want. Think about the thoughts you want to have. If your body tries to tell you it can't keep up, LISTEN to it. All of this to say, when your mouth pops open, rest until you can close your lips again and breathe through your nose. If you do this, you'll get to the point where you can run an entire marathon while nasal breathing if desired.

Ground surface matters and adult knees are bony. If crawling on your hands and knees is painful and it doesn't agree with your knees, you can wear knee pads or crawl on soft, plush surfaces. If that doesn't work, try Commando Crawling on your forearms and thighs.

If hands and knees crawling does not agree with your knees, you can get knee pads or try starting with the Commando Crawl on your forearms and thighs.

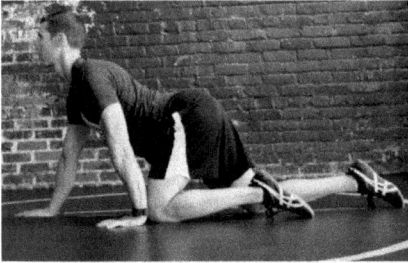

Like this

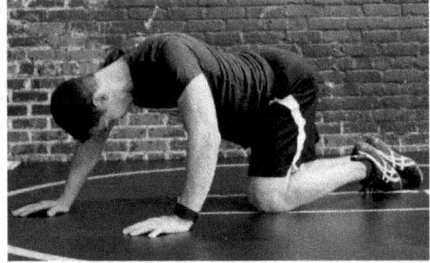

Not like this

- Get on your hands and knees.
- Hold your head up so you can see where you are going.
- Keep a proud chest, like Superman.
- Move your opposite limbs in coordination with each other.
  - The knees should track underneath your body, inside your arms.
- Drag your feet to have more stability. Lift your feet to challenge your stability.
- Keep your tongue on the roof of your mouth!
- Try to maintain breathing through your nose.

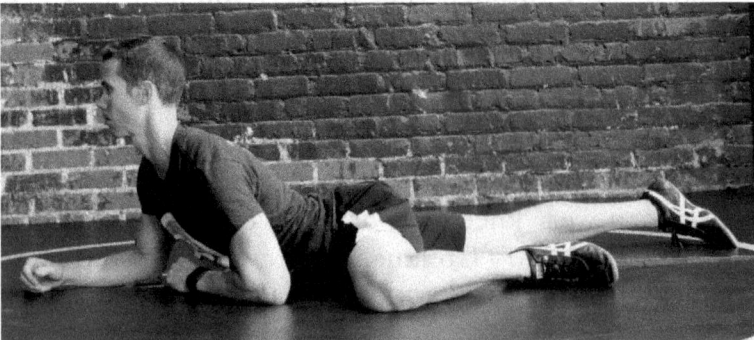

Commando Crawling

Commando Crawling is a regression to hands and knees crawling; it is a way some of us crawl before we push-up on our hands and knees. In the Commando Crawl you crawl on your forearms and your muscular thighs. This makes Commando Crawling a fantastic choice of crawling for those that have tender knees and tender wrists. But just because Commando Crawling is easier on the knees and wrists, and just because it is a regression, that does not mean Commando Crawling is easy. It's not, it's actually quite brutal. It may even help you decide to find some knee pads so you can crawl on your hands and knees.

I like the Commando Crawl for its simplicity. It's almost impossible to do incorrectly and it can be a great "crawling teacher" as it helps people figure out how to use their opposing limbs together. It also encourages and restores mobility in the hips and low back.

I also really like the Commando Crawl for its difficulty. It's just hard to do - it takes a lot of physical effort. But it is a satisfying effort. It allows you to feel reflexive strength happening in your core; it's a great way to discover your abs, probably because it lengthens them and causes them to contract.

Don't overthink it. Just do this:

- Lie on your belly and prop yourself up on your forearms.
- Stay "tall" through your shoulders—do not let your neck sink or sag between your shoulder blades.
- Hold your head up on the horizon.
- Drag your opposite leg in coordination with your opposite arm.
- Keep your tongue on the roof of your mouth.
- Maintain nasal breathing.

Leopard Crawling on the Hands and Feet

After hands and knees crawling has been mastered with a beautiful and fluid crawling pattern in all directions, or after you've built abs of steel with Commando Crawling, you are ready to begin Leopard Crawling on your hands and feet. Leopard Crawling looks very similar to hands and knees crawling in that the head, spine and butt look just as they did when crawling on the hands and knees. The only visible difference is that the knees are elevated off the ground.

After hands and knees crawling has been mastered, and you have a beautiful and fluid crawling pattern in all directions, or after you've built abs of steel with Commando Crawling, you are ready to begin Leopard Crawling on your hands and feet. Leopard Crawling looks very similar to hands and knees crawling in that the head, spine, and butt look just as they did when crawling on the hands and knees. The only visible difference is that the knees are elevated off the ground.

The Leopard Crawling pattern should look fluid and strong, *like* a leopard. It helps to imagine what a leopard looks like when you crawl; it helps the body figure it out.

If I were your strength coach, I'd call Leopard Crawling a progression to the hands and knees crawl and a regression to Spider-man crawling. In the Leopard Crawl, the knees track underneath the body and inside the arms, just as they do when crawling on the hands and knees. This is a great way to crawl in order to build reflexive strength in your center (your X). In fact, it strengthens the center and helps to develop the stability and control needed to perform the Spider-man Crawl.

The Spider-man Crawl requires a higher degree of core muscle coordination and pelvic stability. This is something that is not seen too often in sedentary people. In the absence of this core stability and control, those who attempt to Spider-man Crawl will have very wobbly and uncontrolled hips - their hips will flop from side to side. This could strain the lower back in those with lower back issues.

If you're unsure which crawl to explore, videotape yourself. Wow, remember the videotape? Anyway, if your Leopard Crawl resembles a walking stick more than it does a cat, spend more time crawling on your hands and knees and make that look beautiful. If your Leopard Crawl looks like a beautiful flowing leopard, you can explore the Spider-man Crawl. If your Spider-man crawl looks like a train wreck instead of your friendly neighborhood Spider-man, spend more time in the Leopard Crawl. If your Spider-man and Leopard look beautiful, enjoy them all. They all have their place and are wonderful for you when your body is ready for them.

Remember, be patient, be honest with yourself, and use good judgment.

By the way, just because Leopard Crawling is a regression to Spider-man Crawling does not mean it is easier. Leopard Crawling is much more demanding from a mental and physical standpoint. Leopard Crawling requires many more steps to go the same distance as Spider-man Crawling does. Your legs, hips, core, heart, and lungs will not enjoy it nearly as much as they do Spider-man Crawling!

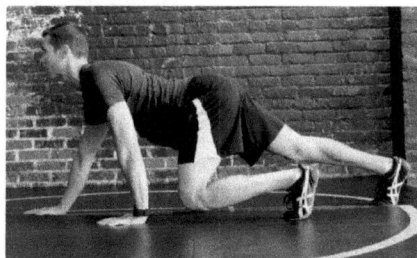

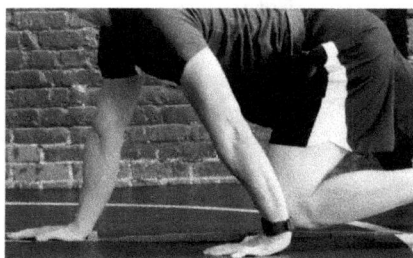

- Get on your hands and feet.
- Hold your eyes and head up on the horizon so that you can see where you are going.
- Keep a proud chest, like Lion-O from the ThunderCats.
- Keep your butt down below your head.
- Do not let your butt rise up above your head.
- Move your opposite limbs in coordination with each other.
- The knees should track underneath your torso, inside your arms.
- In the beginning, it may help to stay long and take small steps with your legs. This helps keep you from overstriding, causing your head to drop and your butt to rise.
- Keep your tongue on the roof of your mouth!
- Try to maintain nasal breathing.

Spider-man Crawling on the Hands and Feet

As mentioned above, Spider-man Crawling is a progression of Leopard Crawling. In the Spider-Man Crawl, the knees will track outside of the torso or outside of the elbows. The head, spine, and butt should remain in the same relationship they did in both the hands and knees crawl and the Leopard Crawl. However, the Spider-man Crawl takes the hips through a much greater range of motion, requiring much more reflexive strength and stability to keep the pelvis level with the ground; it really challenges your rotational stability.

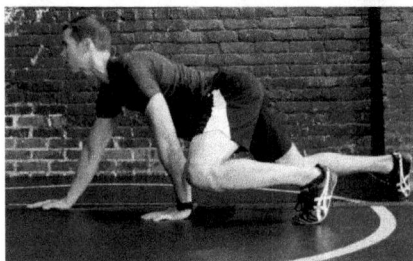

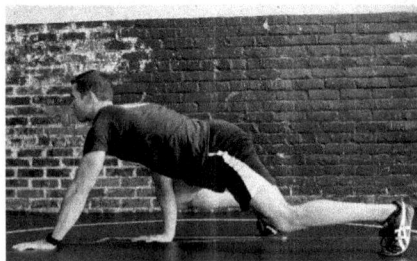

When the body is able to effortlessly handle the demands of this rotational challenge, the body is strong, powerful, and capable.

- Get on your hands and feet.
- Hold your head up so you can see where you are going.
- Keep a proud chest, like Superman (I know, but I love Supes).
- Keep your butt down below your head.
- Do not let your butt rise up above your head.
- Move your opposite limbs in coordination with each other.
- The knees should track outside your arms.
- Keep your tongue on the roof of your mouth!
- Breathe through your nose!

Crawling for Superhuman Strength

Believe it or not, crawling can give you superhuman strength. Actually, you already have superhuman strength inside your body right now; you just don't have access to your strength. Crawling gives you access to your strength potential. It is one of the best ways to really weave the body together—from a physical strength standpoint as well as a neurological health standpoint. You can RESET your body and gain access to your super-strong body simultaneously.

From a traditional "strength training" perspective, Leopard and Spider-man Crawling put more tension on the system. They increase the load and effort required from your body. Done for time or distance, they demand strength. Done consistently, they build strength. One of the reasons these two crawls are so beneficial is they both keep the butt held down below the head while the head is held up. Just holding your body in this position requires tremendous reflexive strength from your core muscles. Every time your hands and feet touch the ground, you reinforce your reflexive strength and dynamic stability by putting pressure on the mechanoreceptors (sensory nerves) in your hands and feet.

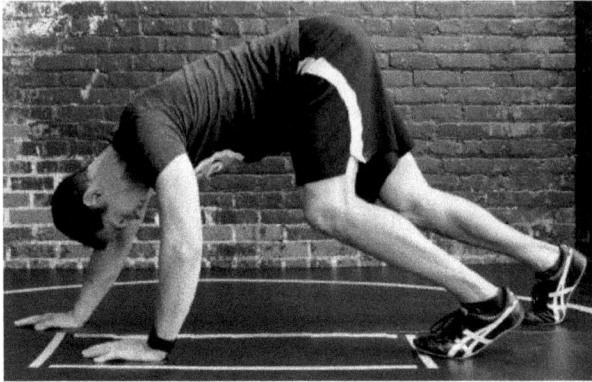

This is not what we want to do. Keep that butt down!

Notice, again, the butt is held down low. This is **not** what we at Original Strength call a "bear crawl." In a bear crawl, the butt is held up, and the head drops down. When this happens, the center of the X is no longer under tension, and the restorative, reflexive postural benefits are lost. Holding the butt down low and keeping the head up on the horizon demands strength from the body's center. In fact, when people tire from Leopard or Spider-man crawling, their butts will pop up like a turkey thermometer.

If the butt pops up, the abs are done, and the turkey is cooked! From a good, better, best movement perspective, bear crawls can be good, but they are not "best" as they leave many benefits on the table. If you're aiming for the most significant performance bang for your buck and you want the optimal expression of your strength, keep your butt down below your head when you crawl.

How can you build a super strong body with crawling?

Simple. Show up often and spend time crawling; practice it and perfect it on a regular basis. If you want to, you can even explore crawling as the only movement in your entire strength training session. If you are adventurous enough to do this, you will be rewarded with a powerful, fluid body. But be warned, crawling for time and/or distance is not as easy as you think it might be initially.

Play around and find out!

Try Leopard or Spider-man crawling for 5 straight minutes and evaluate your experience. How did you do? Were you able to keep your lips shut? Were you able to hold your head up? Did your butt pop up? Did you have to stop and rest?

If you tried this, you likely noticed that crawling takes strength, stamina, a good heart, and great lungs. It works ALL of YOU. It builds all of you, too.

Crawling builds all the physical qualities you want to have, especially if you hold your tongue on the roof of your mouth and breathe in and out of your nose while you crawl. This is not easy to do, but it can become easy over time. If you show up to crawl often enough, eventually, you'll get really good at crawling. This means that you will be really good at expressing your strength and power.

But there is more to crawling than just the benefit of gaining physical expression. There's also the tenacity aspect, or the "I am able" aspect of crawling. It develops your "I can-ness."

Crawling on the hands and feet for any appreciable distance or time is really hard to do. It sucks. At least until it doesn't. And that's the point.

We often ask people, "If you could Leopard Crawl for 10 straight minutes without stopping, what can you not do?"

The answer is, "You can do anything you want to do."

Why?

Because you would be as strong as you want to be, in both mind and body. Crawling builds whole strength. It is extremely diffi-cult on the mind to crawl for time or distance because it is so physically demanding. It's miserable. When you get to the point that you can crawl for 10 straight minutes without stopping, you have gotten to the point where you have overcome the physical and mental miserableness of crawling.

You have the ability to do hard things, to tackle and overcome mental and physical obstacles. It helps you to develop willpower, tenacity, grit, strength, stamina, focus, ability, and "I can-ness." There isn't much you cannot endure and conquer when you can fluidly crawl on your hands and feet for 10 straight minutes.

Please understand that I'm not recommending you crawl for 10 minutes. I'm only alluding to the possibility that you are capable of doing so. If you ever discover that for yourself, you'll discover that you're quite capable of almost anything else because you'll know "I can."

Just say that in your mind and notice how it feels.

"I can."

Crawling builds this knowledge. And this is the knowledge that makes life better.

Anyway, your body already has everything inside of it that you could ever need to become powerful, strong, and resilient. You are never stuck or limited. To become unlimited, explore and practice crawling. When your body is ready, you can progress your crawling by increasing time, distance or both. You can also practice crawling in multiple directions (forward, backward, sideways, in circles…) and by changing speeds. You can even add resistance to your crawling by adding weight to your body or dragging things while you crawl.

You don't need a room full of weights, machines, or gadgets to build strength. You can crawl. The best thing is that crawling has very few barriers to entry. You can do it anywhere, no matter where you are. It is low-skill; the program lives inside of you. It's not even dangerous. Heck, if you fall, you're already on the ground! The point is that you were made to crawl, and crawling is the movement that was intended to make you strong.

Again, if you want to express your full strength potential, make room for crawling in your life. Any of the ways I've mentioned here are great. I will say that Leopard and Spider-Man crawling look super cool (to me), and they both build ridiculous strength, but don't dismiss crawling on your hands and knees.

Crawling on your hands and knees will still give you access to your strength potential. It's not as hard as crawling on your hands and feet, but the benefits to your brain and your body are still there. Many days, I only practice crawling on my hands and knees. It feels terrific and allows me to explore the movement and discover things about my body that I would miss if I didn't do it. Crawling on my hands and knees is where I learn how to move and how to feel the connections of my strength and control. It's a movement goldmine.

The point is, do not miss the powerful simplicity of this beautiful movement. It will give you access to yourself, allowing you to achieve your expression potential. It doesn't really matter how you crawl, just crawl—often.

Yes, people will stare. That does not matter. Crawl anyway. Strength is not afraid, it is courageous. Besides, giving the neighbors something to talk about is really fun. But more than that, it's really empowering to know "I can."

To learn more about crawling and its variations, here is a crawling playlist:

https://www.youtube.com/
playlist?list=PL9v3pv_KGM7sin0JMX-7BPGrsyxx4iQ67

I Climbed a Mountain

"I climbed a mountain this year. Something I didn't think I would be able to do again, and I owe it in large part to Original Strength and one of their trainers, Trevor Trebbien.

I have been a massage therapist for about 22 years. Have learned and taught about movement and how to take care of one's self for many years. Due to my own history and background, I've always loved taking care of others; it was always easier than taking care of myself.

By the time I realized all the activities I wasn't doing any more like hiking, dancing, or even walking much, my body decided it was time to make me pay attention. 2 years ago, my right hip literally gave out on me. Long story short, it changed everything. After a visit to the ER and learning I had severe arthritis to the point of holes in my bones and nothing left for cushion in the joints, both hips got replaced within 6 weeks of each other. One surgery went really well, and one did not. I couldn't walk, work, or even go back to my own home due to not being able to navigate stairs, and I wasn't even 50 yet.

As great as my Physical therapists were, they had gone as far as they could, and I still needed something more. Discovering a Cross Fit Groupon coupon, I decided to try Trevor's gym, and once again, everything in my life was about to change, this time for the better.

When I learned about the Pressing RESET method and the key part about learning to crawl, I had no idea of the far-reaching implications it would have. The spark created by re-patterning my body and brain to move forward in a healthy way started to seep into every part of my being and how I chose to live.

Through the Original Strength work and the help of Trevor and his staff, I gained a life that I had almost forgotten about. I learned that I could be strong again.

Re-patterning and learning to crawl has become a mantra for my mental, emotional, and spiritual well-being as well. It was a key for me that unlocked my life. I realized I could go from crawling to moving forward to climbing mountains.

It doesn't get better than that as far as I'm concerned, and I am so grateful."

—Corrine Ranard
Portland Oregon

DO THIS ONE THING. FOREVER.

"There is another."
–Yoda, Empire Strikes Back

As powerful as crawling can be, it is not the most potent RESET. There is another. That designation is reserved for cross-crawls. Cross-crawls are the simplest, most powerful movements that anyone can do. They are the simplest because nearly anyone can do them regardless of physical condition. They are the most powerful for the very same reason; anyone can do them. And at the speed of anyone's nervous system, Cross-crawls can restore hope. They make everything better instantly.

Cross-crawls are performed by simply touching opposite limbs together. To do this, you have to cross the midline of your body and touch your opposite leg somewhere with your opposite hand or arm. You've likely performed Cross-crawls before, maybe when you were a child in P.E. class or when you participated in warm-ups during team sports practices.

For those of us who did them, Cross-crawls were more than likely simply a movement we used very briefly to prepare for other physical activities. We did them to "warm up," but we didn't really know their benefits. Let me just say that Cross-crawls are so much more than just a movement used to warm the body up for athletic endeavors.

In the world of brain development and rehabilitation, Cross-crawls have long been used to treat learning disabilities in children as well as help stroke patients regain their normal function. Can you imagine the wonder of this movement? Simply touching the right hand to the left leg and touching the left hand to the right leg has the power and potential to create new neural connections in a damaged or compromised brain and restore function to a person's body. That's pretty much miraculous, no matter how you look at it.

Remember, crossing the body's midline, and performing Cross-crawls has many of the same brain-building benefits as crawling. This means Cross-crawls share many of the same physical benefits as crawling does. This is because the neural benefits from Cross-crawls lead to better access to the body's expressions. Cross-crawls can help a person regain their body.

Why are Cross-crawls the most powerful RESET?

Because anyone, regardless of their physical condition, can perform some type of Cross-crawl. Not everyone can get down on the floor and crawl around. Not everyone will be able to remember how to use their diaphragm when they breathe. But anyone and everyone can perform a Cross-crawl. And when they do, miracles can and do happen.

Nearly all the Original Strength Coaches could offer an incredible true story of the power of Cross-crawls. We've all had encounters with the wonder of this movement.

We've seen some wild things. For example, we have seen people who were unable to stand from a chair on their own, stand up, unassisted, after learning how to perform Cross-crawls.

We've seen people go from needing a walker or a cane to walking without the aid of their device after learning how to do Cross-crawls within seconds of performing the Cross-crawls. Because of this, we've even seen a husband get his wife back at the speed of her nervous system once she performed the Cross-crawls. What I mean is that a man witnessed vitality and strength return to his wife's body within seconds of learning how to perform Cross-crawls. He watched her walk away unassisted for the first time in a long time.

I know that sounds unbelievable, but it is undoubtedly true, and that is what a true RESET does. It improves and can even restore function at the speed of the nervous system. Cross-crawls make an impact as soon as they are done, regardless of whether the effect is witnessed or not. They work from the inside out.

Cross-crawls are the simplest, most powerful, most accessible, and most restorative RESET there is. It is the most accessible because anyone can do it. It is the most powerful because of the hope it can give a person. Cross-crawls can change a person's life by restoring their life. And that is why, regardless of your health and condition, you should consider performing Cross-crawls every single day, forever.

They are too simple and too powerful not to do. I've done at least 20 Cross-crawl touches nearly every day now for over 10 years. I plan to do them for the rest of my life.

Focusing With Your Tongue

Another nice benefit of performing Cross-crawls is that they increase focus and mental alertness; they can help remove mental fogginess and fight away the sleep monster. If you can't find a cup of coffee, you can always enjoy a quick Cross-crawl movement snack.

Speaking of mental alertness, the position of your tongue can also increase mental alertness. The tongue stimulates the vestibular system and activates the RAS (the Reticular Activating System), increasing focus and balance.[41] The RAS is responsible for regulating arousal and sleep-wake transitions in people. Holding the tongue on the roof of your mouth, and even pressing the tongue against the roof of your mouth, can stimulate the RAS system and make you more alert and able to focus. This is also like a "wake up" movement snack when you can't make that instant cup of coffee. It's a mental alertness RESET!

So, combining Cross-crawls with pressing your tongue on the roof of your mouth could be that nice mental spark you need to be more productive, more creative, and more alert. The next time you need to concentrate, focus, remember, or be on your A-game, stand up, press your tongue against the roof of your mouth, and perform 20 big-motioned Cross-crawls. Notice how you feel and notice how you perform. Then tell your friends.

Any Which Way You Can

I know I just told you to stand up and perform 20 big-motioned Cross-crawls, but Cross-crawls can be performed in almost any position that you can put your body into. They can be performed in a chair, on the floor while lying on your back, standing, walking, or even skipping.

Traditionally, Cross-crawls are done standing by touching the opposite elbow to the opposite knee. This requires both a bit of balance and mobility. However, it is not the only way.

If you cannot touch your opposite elbow to your opposite knee, simply touch your opposite hand or forearm to your opposite knee or thigh. If you do not have the balance to perform the Cross-crawl while standing, try them lying down on your back. You can even perform Cross-crawl sit-ups like Rocky Balboa if you want to. No matter your abilities or physical limitations, you should be able to find a way to perform a Cross-crawl.

Cross-crawls can also easily be progressed to more challenging versions. For instance, if you have no trouble touching your elbow to your knee while standing, try performing Cross-crawls while you keep your fingertips behind your ears. If keeping your fingertips behind your ears is easy, try doing that with your eyes closed or with your eyes looking in the opposite direction of where you are rotating. Try Cross-crawling while marching forward, try them while marching backward, try them super-slow, try them while skipping or even while skipping and spinning around in circles. You can even try them in the rain and on a train! With or without green eggs and ham…

All combinations and variations of Cross-crawls are good and beneficial. Do what you can. It really doesn't matter *how* you do them as much as it matters *that* you do them.

They can be done anywhere: at work, the grocery store, the gym, the elevator, the men's room, or anywhere. On second thought, all variations of Cross-crawls may be beneficial, but all locations for performing them may not. If you do decide to do them in the restroom, make sure it is a private restroom.

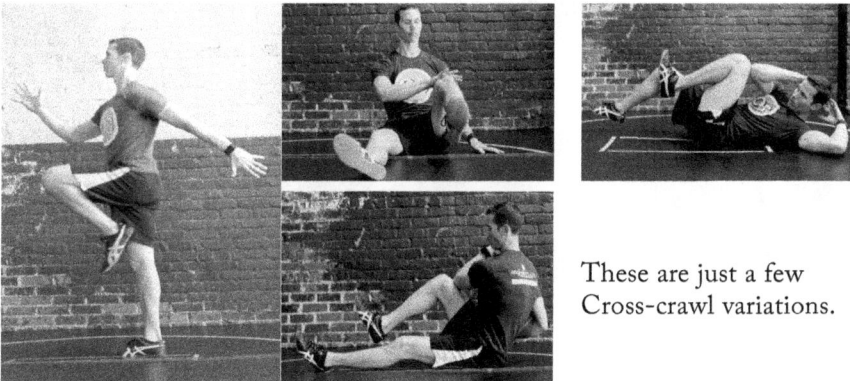

These are just a few Cross-crawl variations.

Performing Cross-Crawls

- Cross-crawls can be done in any position.
- Touch your opposite elbow to your opposite knee.
- If your mobility does not allow you to touch your opposite elbow to your opposite knee, you can touch your opposite hand or forearm to your opposite knee or thigh.

> The most innocent-looking movement

- Explore various ways in which you can touch your opposite limbs together.
- For extra benefit, perform them slowly unless you are skipping.
- Keep your tongue on the roof of your mouth and breathe through your nose!

Remember, do not dismiss the power of the Cross-crawl. This is perhaps the most innocent-looking movement, but it could have the most powerful impact on you or your loved ones.

Do yourself a favor. Perform Cross-crawls every single day.

One Touch at a Time

"*In using the Original Strength RESETS, we have found that adding Cross-crawls, even while sitting, will help to reinforce the balance and coordination gains we are making in therapy. It is safe, can be easily made more or less challenging, and isn't physically taxing to the patient.*

In the clinic, we have seen some of the most drastic improvements in patients who have Parkinson's disease. **Parkinson's is a progressive disorder of the nervous system that affects movement.** *It often affects walking, balance, coordination, and speech. As Parkinson's disease progresses, so do the symptoms. The hope, with therapy, is to slow down the progression and maintain the status quo.* **Improvement is not much of a consideration.** *However, with the addition of Cross-crawls, even while sitting, we have seen patients improve with their standardized balance testing.*

Barbara is an 85-year-old female with a history of back and knee pain. Late in 2014, she was diagnosed with Parkinson's. 'I was very troubled by what I heard when I got my diagnosis. Along with my concern of falling, I was worried I would no longer be able to continue coordinating ministry here in my community or enjoy activities with my friends.'

Her initial Tinetti score was 7/28, a 75% disability. Her most recent Tinetti Balance score was 21/28, an improvement of 300%! All while having a progressive disease where maintaining physical skill is considered success and advancement is rare. There have been no changes in medication and very few changes in her therapy program from her previous interactions with physical therapists, except for Pressing Reset with Cross-crawling both in therapy and at home. Barbara is pleased with both the physical progress and the emotional response. 'Not only does it seem to work, but it is also easy, and I can work on it on my own. I have some control again; not many 85 year olds can say that."

–Chris Stulginsky, PT
Charlotte, NC

FOUR LEGS GOOD, TWO LEGS BETTER!

If you've ever read George Orwell's *Animal Farm*, you know four legs are good, but ultimately, two legs are better. As humans, we are indeed made to live and move through the majority of our lives on two feet. In fact, we were designed to consistently "Press RESET" moment by moment through our gait pattern. Walking was intended to be the movement that keeps our brains and bodies tied together. Every step we take *should* be a neurological and physical RESET. But that is not necessarily the case because many of us have missed a step.

If crawling was meant to be the *foundation* of our gait pattern—and it was—then walking was meant to be the *structure* from which we move. We were designed to walk in strength, with strength, and towards strength. Our gait patterns weave us and hold us together. They nourish our brains and prepare us to transfer powerful forces throughout our bodies. At least, that was the plan.

But, let's be honest, how much walking do you really do? And when you do walk, do you feel strength flowing through your body? You should.

Since man began, man has been extremely strong and resilient. He built amazing structures like pyramids and coliseums—with his brain and his body. There were no machines. There were no bulldozers, no earthmovers, no Ford F-150s, and no cars. There were camels, horses, donkeys, oxen, and men. Brilliant and resilient men with strong backs and legs of steel. Their bodies were made out of iron. They moved, they worked, and they walked. Almost everywhere they went, they went on foot, and more than likely, every step they took was a step of restoration.

Yes, they had sicknesses, germs, and diseases but also capability and resiliency. They were strong, and they were fit for the tasks at hand. There is a reason Michelangelo could sculpt a beautiful, muscular statue like David. He saw men that looked like that. It would be hard to pull such a sculpture out of your imagination if your eyes only knew brokenness.

The point is that man was made to walk, and man was made for strength.

Fast forward a couple thousand years. Today, most of us don't walk so much. And when we do, we are not necessarily walking in our design. We are not standing tall with good posture. We are not swinging our arms from our shoulders. Half the time, most of us don't even swing our arms. Instead, we slouch, look down at the ground, look down at our smartphones, or keep our hands in our pockets. We are not walking *deliberately* with purpose, the way we were made to walk. Man is not being *man*.

Now, think about a lion. They are beautiful, strong, and graceful because they act like lions. They do what they were created to do. What I mean by *walking with purpose* is that we should walk like the pinnacle of creations we are - human beings. We should walk around as if we owned the world, with tall postures, holding our heads up on the horizon, swinging our arms from our shoulders. When we walk, it should look like power, grace, and poetry. In fact, the rest of the world's animals should stop what they are doing and watch us move as we walk because we should be the most beautiful moving creatures on the planet.

But today, because of our lifestyles, walking is not the RESET it was intended to be. As a consequence, we are not as well connected and tied together as we were meant to be. This is what makes crawling so powerful. It is foundational in that it weaves us back together.

Start walking intentionally as you begin Pressing RESET and exploring the ideas I've shared thus far. When you walk, walk deliberately. Instead of ambling on two legs, walk with purpose using four limbs. Swing your arms from your shoulders. Allow your shoulders and hips to work together like they do when you crawl. Stand tall. Keep a long spine like you do when you are rocking. Keep the crown of your head pointing towards the sky. Don't worry; this will become virtually automatic the more you engage in the rest of the RESETS.

Seriously, make time in your day to start taking purposeful walks. Not only can this be a resetting, cross-lateral exercise, but it can also be mentally freeing and rejuvenating. Walking can set things right. It removes stress, nourishes our brains, frees creativity, gives us clarity, and gives us access to our strength. Walking is intended to be *THE RESET we were always meant to do.*

"But we have risen and stand upright."
—Psalm 20:8

Arm Yourself

Maybe the pigs in Orwell's *Animal Farm* were really right from the beginning: "Four legs good, two legs bad." As I said above, we are designed to use all four limbs when walking and running. This is imperative for our overall health and ability to retain our original strength as we age.

Using your arms when you walk keeps your brain healthy. It takes the right side of your brain to swing your left arm, and it takes the left side of your brain to swing your right arm. Swinging your right arm nourishes the left side of your brain, and swinging your left arm nourishes the right side of your brain. Again, movement and brain health have a very *chicken-and-egg* relationship. They both create and sustain each other.

Here is why this is so important. Brain deterioration in adults is correlated with the deterioration of balance.[42] When elderly people start to lose their balance, their gait widens to increase their stability and reduce their chance of falling. Their arms also barely swing if they swing at all. But why does their brain deteriorate? Why does their balance start to go away? Which one happens first? Is it because they don't swing their arms? Maybe. Is it because they are more sedentary than they used to be? Probably. Whatever the reason, many of the typical aging woes can be mitigated, if not prevented, if we live and move in our design. We are designed to swing our arms when we walk. Swinging our arms from the shoulders keeps the brain healthy.

Look around you. How many people do you see who swing their arms from their shoulders when they walk? You may see an elbow swing, or you may see a sway from the spine, or you may simply see no arm movement at all. In all of these people who don't move their arms, their brains are not getting the full nourishment it was designed to have from walking.

60 Minutes, the CBS news show, ran a documentary titled, "Living to 90 and Beyond".[43] It was fascinating. They revealed some interesting commonalities shared by those who live past 90. They also pondered why some of those who lived over 90 years of age had no signs of brain dementia or Alzheimer's Disease while others did. It turns out that just because you live past 90 years of age doesn't guarantee that you won't get Alzheimer's Disease. The point is that they followed the 90-plus-year-olds around on camera, and there was a fascinating characteristic that the non-Alzheimer 90-year-olds shared: they swung their arms when they walked. The others with Alzheimer's did not swing their arms. This is just my observation, not the reporting staff of *60 Minutes*. But still, it makes you wonder.

Let's extrapolate. Crawling, the foundation of our gait pattern is composed of four moving limbs. Therefore, walking, our predominant gait pattern, should be an expression of four moving limbs. I think this is why marching is such a powerful RESET; it is very deliberate in that it requires all four limbs to contra-laterally mirror one another. In fact, I refer to marching as crawling while standing.

How to Crawl on Two Feet

Marching is a very powerful RESET. When done properly, it coordinates the hips *and* shoulders together, much like crawling. Basically, it is crawling on two feet.

Like Cross-crawls, marching has all the benefits of crawling. It is also a great RESET for mental alertness and improves overall physical performance. One thing that marching does better than crawling is that marching moves the shoulders into extension. (NOTE: Crawling moves the shoulders towards extension but cannot move the shoulders past the plane of the torso. Marching extends the shoulders beyond and past the torso.) When we march, the shoulders are deliberately swung from flexion to extension and vice versa. It feels quite pleasant, even wonderful when the arms extend beyond the torso. There is something very therapeutic about the arms swinging into extension.

And it is the extension part that is so important. Not only does it feel amazing, but when you consider that our opposite limbs are actually supposed to mirror each other when we walk and run, the idea of shoulder extension becomes a big deal. In our gait pattern, our opposing limbs should move and swing together in rhythm with relatively the same range of motion. If the shoulders are not swinging or are not fully used during walking or running, will the hips be able to move through their full range of motion with full power?

In other words, how effective or efficient is our stride when we walk if our shoulders are not moving through their intended range of motion? Could this be a contributing factor or THE reason people get "sleepy glutes" because their shoulders never move into extension when they walk? What if low back and hip problems could be alleviated by fully engaging in our design to walk - swinging the shoulders to match the hips? The mirroring motion of our limbs is important.

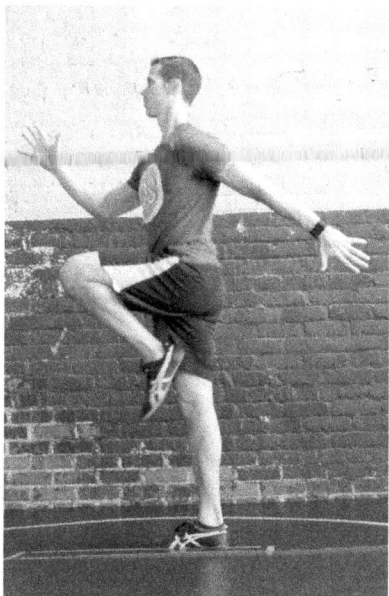

Notice how the opposite limbs mirror each other. The opposite elbow and knee both go into flexion on cross-pattern, while the other elbow and knee both go into extension. The same thing happens in the opposite shoulders and hips. They mirror each other.

Tim is actually marching in place here, but do you see the shoulder extension?

This is one of the reasons marching is so powerful. It resets shoulder extension, which could mean improving and resetting hip extension as well. This means marching can help restore walking to the apex RESET it is intended to be.

Another benefit of marching is that it can also help prepare the body for generating and transferring incredible amounts of force. After all, it's just a hop away from skipping. Marching helps weave the body together and can prepare the body's tissues for expression of power.

How many people do you know who decide to go from living a sedentary life for ten years to desiring to run a 5K at the flip of a switch? Ever heard of the "From Couch to 5k" program? This may not be the best idea if the body hasn't been prepared for all the forces that running generates. In fact, I can tell you without hesitation that a couch cannot and will not prepare anyone for those kinds of forces.

But marching can. Marching can be an easy, "gentle" way to prepare the body for the forces running generates. It can help strengthen and reinforce the feet, ankles, calves, knees, hips, and tendons! When marching, it is easy to vary the intensity of how much force you put into the ground and the speed at which you do it. This prepares the body's "springs," the Achilles tendons, and gastroc muscles, to leap and bound across the ground. If you march fast enough, you may even notice that you want to run. It is not unusual for people to report that a desire to break into a sprint comes over them when they practice marching. Friends, this is a GOOD feeling. Marching taps into a hidden desire in your design—the desire to fly, sprint, and experience the ultimate expression of your movement design.

How to March:

Marching can be done in a variety of ways, but I prefer the following method:

- Drive your arms from your shoulders and ensure they move from front to back.

- Really focus on driving the arms back into extension.
- The opposite arm should drive forward as the opposite knee drives upward.
- Plant and push off of the balls of your feet when marching. NO heel striking.
- The rise of the knees should match the range of motion and drive of the arms.
- The arms and legs should move crisply together.
- The fingers should be spread wide.

It is easy to transition from marching to skipping. Skipping is a RESET. It combines the movement of marching with a rhythmic hop. Like marching, skipping is a great way to prepare the body to absorb and transfer force. It also teaches the body how to "land" from the small jumps skipping employs.

The cross-lateral, rhythmic, gentle bounding of skipping taps into another hidden quality buried inside your design: Joy. You have probably never witnessed an angry child or a sad adult skipping. Instead, if you've ever watched someone skip, you have witnessed an unmistakable joy in their facial expression and body movements. Joy is tied to our movements. When we move well, when we move as we should, it brings out the joy inside of us. If you don't believe me, go for a skip. I challenge you not to feel good while you do it.

Remember, everything about you is connected; you are whole. How you move is tied to how you feel. You were clearly designed to move, so you were clearly designed for joy. You were made to feel good AND to experience joy. There is no way around this simple truth.

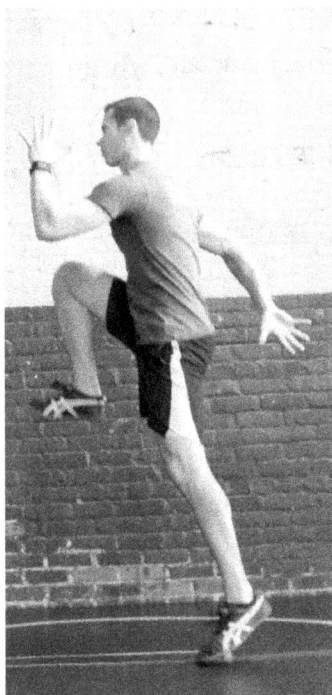

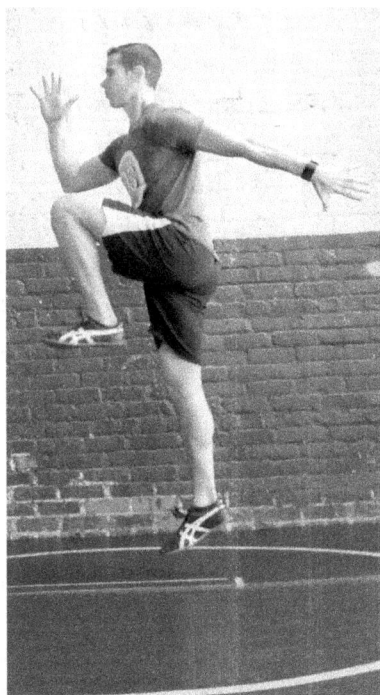

Again, skipping is just like marching with a rhythmic hop in each step.

How to Skip:

- Skipping can also be done in a variety of ways, but I still prefer the following method:
- Drive your arms from your shoulders and ensure they move from front to back.
- Really focus on driving the arms back into extension.
- The opposite arm should drive forward as the opposite knee drives upward, lifting your body off the ground.
- Plant and push off of the balls of your feet when skipping.
- Land and absorb the impact on the ground with the balls of the feet as well. NO heel striking.

- The rise of the knees should match the range of motion and the drive of the arms.
- The arms and legs should move crisply together.
- The fingers should be spread wide.

Express Yourself

Sprinting is the ultimate expression of human design. It is the simultaneous display of speed, power, grace, fluidity, strength, and beauty. There is nothing more beautiful than a well-connected sprinting body in motion. Just as we were made to walk, we were also made to sprint.

Sprinting is a RESET. Unless it's not… But it should be. After all, it is a progression of crawling and walking. It is a movement that should help nourish the brain and keep the body well-connected. And it can if the body has a solid foundation of reflexive strength.

When we live in our design and move the way we were designed to move and are well prepared to sprint, sprinting becomes a RESET. It helps build reflexive strength at a higher level of force. Sprinting prepares our bodies to explode: To create, absorb, and transfer high forces at high speeds. In other words, sprinting can help prepare us for life and all the physical impacts and demands it throws at us. There was a time in man's history when sprinting was likely our highest survival mechanism. It got us out of danger and helped us witness another day.

But we can't live in the past! Depending on your present physical condition, the idea of sprinting may be a bit outlandish to you. But entertain the possibility that somewhere inside of you, there is a sprinter. However, you may not be ready to wake your inner sprinter up just yet. Because of its demands, the powerful nature of sprinting, and the forces it generates, you want to make sure your body is prepared to sprint should you ever decide to sprint.

You need a solid foundation to handle the beautiful power sprinting generates.

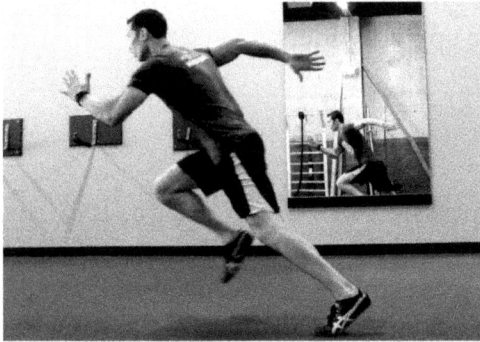

How do you do this? The same way you did as a child. You spend some time Pressing RESET and exploring all the other RESETS I've discussed to this point. You recreate a solid foundation of reflexive strength, the solid foundation that you once had as a child. You will be ready to sprint once you have tied your body back together.

A word of caution:

If you do fancy the idea of sprinting and you want to try it, BE PATIENT. When you are ready when you have Pressed RESET enough times and tied your X together, "play" with sprinting. "Play" means to *explore*. Explore what sprinting is like; be curious, but don't be aggressive.

Get great at crawling. Then, get great at marching. Then, get really good at skipping. Learn how to march and skip gently. Learn how to march and skip powerfully. This can help prepare you and ease yourself into sprinting. When ready, you can sprint at **half-speed** and work your way up to three-quarter speed. When half-speed and three-quarter speed start feeling good, you may be ready for full speed! But again, BE PATIENT and work your way up to this over time. It may take days, weeks, or months before you are ready. That's okay. It is a process. Enjoy the process.

Restoring Your Feet

While we are on the topic of sprinting, this is a good time to discuss the importance of healthy feet. Believe it or not, *you were born without shoes*. Yes, it is true. When you came into the world, your feet were bare. They were perfectly made to grasp the ground and develop into a solid platform on which you would stand. Feet, much like the hands, are full of nerve endings that send proprioceptive information to your brain. The nerves in your feet help paint a picture in your brain of where your body is and what it is doing. They help build a clear, complete movement map in your brain, and they should inform the brain of how and when to fire the muscles in your legs.

If your brain is getting optimal information from all the sensory nerves in your feet, from the skin, joints and muscles, your movement map will be clear and you will move optimally. If your brain is not getting optimal information from your feet, your movement map will be "fuzzy", or less clear and your movements may be inhibited. This is where shoes can limit our potential. Did you know shoes can distort the information your brain receives from your feet? Yep, that's why you were born without them.

Your feet are two highly sensory-rich platforms that reflexively engage your body. They are designed to support your weight, produce and absorb force, and feed your brain with the information needed to initiate the appropriately timed, reflexive responses you need to stand, walk, run, and jump. In his book *Power to The People*, Pavel Tsatsouline points out, "…another power boosting reflex is called the positive support reaction. This reflex causes the leg musculature to contract in response to the pressure on the sole of the foot."[44] Pavel goes on to mention the *extensor reflex*, which causes the leg muscles to fire in a precise pattern depending on how the foot hits the ground.[45] This means there is a rhythm, a sequence of reflexive firing, that happens in the body's musculature dependent on how the foot touches and feels the ground.

Wearing shoes that restrict the motion of the feet and blunt their contact with the ground due to the thick, cushiony soles would be like wearing an oven mitt on your hands. It robs you of your full dexterity and diminishes your sense of feeling. This slows your reflexes and inhibits your strength, as your brain is not able to get a clear picture of what your body is doing. The brain needs to receive clear signals to respond with optimal reflexive actions and reactions when needed.

Another problem with wearing shoes all the time is that some shoes are made to mimic the job of the foot, removing the need for the foot to fulfill its design. For example, If a shoe has a supporting arch, why does the brain need to support the muscles created to give the foot its natural arch? Remember the SAID Principle. The body adapts to what it does and operates on the "use it or lose it" rule. If you don't need to use your arch, you won't. This is how you can lose it.

Please understand that I'm not against wearing shoes. My wife would tell you I have a shoe problem; she thinks I have way too many pairs. I do love shoes. And I wear them when the conditions call for protecting my feet. That, and being barefoot in a restaurant, seems to be frowned upon. But when I can, I do go barefoot and try to spend a good deal of time being barefoot. I also wear "minimalist" shoes or "barefoot" shoes 99% of the time when I do wear shoes. After all, I want strong, healthy feet. That is the point: if your goal is to become as resilient as possible, it may be a good idea to spend some time barefooted, especially when you train.

The feet are the foundation of our upright existence. Healthy feet are essential *and foundational* to a healthy body. If you want to truly optimize and restore your original strength, you need to restore your feet as well.

Ponder this. Each foot has 26 bones, 33 joints, and more than 100 muscles, tendons, and ligaments. There are also sensory nerves throughout these joints, muscles, and tendons. These joints were made to move, and these muscles and tendons were made to support you and your life activities.

The feet are our connection with the ground and our base of support. They are designed to be among the strongest, most resilient parts of our body. They are our roots; the strength and resilience of the feet grant strength and resilience to the body.

CAUTION:

If you have spent years in shoes (what some people refer to as foot coffins), ease into going barefoot. Don't try to run a 5K barefoot your first time without shoes. Trust me on this. I did that for you so that you would not have to. It took me about three weeks to be able to walk like a normal person again. If the wind were to blow the hairs on my calves, it would hurt like crazy. I'll say it again. DO NOT try to run a 5K the day you decide to go barefoot. Ease into it. Spend some time at home simply walking around barefoot. Get used to walking on different surfaces. Feel the various surfaces and the information your feet provide.

A great way to ease into being barefoot is to spend time Pressing RESET without shoes. Rocking and crawling are phenomenal ways to introduce all those wonderful joints in your feet to movement. Suppose you are strong enough to crawl on your hands and feet. In that case, Leopard or Spider-man crawling is another excellent way to strengthen your feet as they do not place the full weight of your body on your feet. Hmm… It is kind of like learning how to crawl before you walk.

If you go back to the beginning in your body, you will be able to reach the ending you desire. Spend time restoring your feet. Spend time Pressing RESET. It is well worth it, and you won't be disappointed.

THE GUIDE TO PRESSING RESET

So now you know the RESETS, the Big 5 movements you were born to do. These are the movements that can help you live your life better. In truth, there are many variations to these 5 movements, more than I could ever list in a book.

The variations to these movements may be smaller or easier to perform breakdowns of the RESETS. These could be called regressions. They can also be bigger, more challenging versions as well. These could be called progressions. Do not let this overwhelm you. There are still only 5 RESETS to focus on. These five RESETS are our foundational movement patterns, the movements upon which our lives are meant to be built.

To review, they are:

- Proper nasal and diaphragmatic breathing
- Building head control via moving the eyes and the head
- Rolling
- Rocking
- Crawling/Cross-crawling/Gait patterns

Play with and explore the easier versions I've listed above for now. When you think you understand those and want to explore the rest, feel free to do so. Remember, there is no algorithm or magic combination to Pressing RESET. Engaging in the Big 5, even if it seems too easy and too simple, is Pressing RESET on your body. It can restore your original strength. You can become as resilient and strong as you have ever wanted to be just by spending a few minutes exploring these movements every day.

The Numerics of Neurology

Your brain and nervous system are established through repetition or lack of it. They follow the "use it or lose it" principle. If you don't use your body, your brain will prune away the pathways you no longer use. The brain strives to be energy efficient and it is very cost conscious. It takes energy to keep neural pathways we are not using, so the brain removes them if they aren't used. This is one of the wonders of our design. Our body basically gives us what we ask of it through use.

This really means that the "use it or lose it" principle is the "use it to build it and keep it" principle. We get to co-create our nervous system through movement and thought. And we do that through engagement. If we want something from our body, we ask for it by engaging in the very thing we want. If we keep showing up to move every day, we ask the brain to always be able to move. In an effort to become energy efficient, the brain will start to build neural pathways, like neural superhighways, that allow us to access the qualities we want.

For example, when you make a movement, you create a neural pathway for that movement.[46] If you keep making that movement, you engrave that neural pathway in your brain. Once the pathway is engraved (myelinated), it becomes a very efficient pathway that allows you to make that movement quickly, effortlessly, and often subconsciously. This is how habits are created through repetition. The body is made to adapt to what it does. Remember the SAID principle (Specific Adaptation to Imposed Demand)—it states that the body will adapt to the stresses that are placed on it.[47]

Conversely, when you don't make a movement, perhaps a movement you used to make, your body eventually starts pruning those neural connections associated with that specific movement. This is called neural pruning.[48] When you were a teenager, you underwent a massive neural pruning. Your brain removed many of the unused neural connections in your brain that you were no longer using to prepare you for the ones you would be making as an adult. It was kind of like a "spring cleaning" for your brain.

Adults also experience neural pruning from lack of use. Not moving and not performing specific movements weaken the neural connections in the brain for those movements. If they are not totally removed, those connections become "dull," weak, and less efficient. Essentially, you can starve your neural pathways through disuse, but you can also feed them through use.

There are other consequences to not engaging in your design. Not only does it weaken the neural connections between your brain and your body, but it also weakens the tissues in your body as well. Movement stimulates and builds your muscles, tendons, ligaments, and fascia because you are using them. The "stress" of movement requires the body to nourish these tissues with oxygen, energy, nutrients, and so on.

Lack of movement is a lack of stress on the body's tissues. This results in atrophy. The body will not keep what it does not need. Or, from the SAID principle perspective, if there is no demand placed on the body, there is no adaptation to maintain. Another way to look at it is that if you are demanding nothing, you will get nothing.

And that's the point - the body adapts. Whether you do or do not do, the brain and body will accommodate you through adaptation. Now, consider that you were actually designed to Press RESET throughout the day every day of your life. You were born Pressing RESET, moving, and living through the Big 5 movements. This is what wove your brain and body together through healthy neural connections and healthy tissues.

What happens if we don't live in that design? What happens if we trade our movement for a stationary living?

We prune ourselves away.

The neural connections in our brain, the foundations of our movement vocabulary, get weaker and less efficient. At the same time, our body adapts through atrophy, weakness, immobility, and poor posture. And because how we move affects how we feel, we get weaker and frail, and our soul shrinks as well. We become anxious, fearful, stressed out, agitated, self-absorbed, insecure, and emotionally unstable. Our whole being shrinks and atrophies. We are not designed for this. This is not the way.

I do love our modern world. I cannot imagine being born in another time. The technologies, foods, and luxuries we get to experience are true blessings. But with our modern world there is less of a need for us to live in our design to move. In fact, our current world distracts us and hinders us from moving due to our conveniences, advancements, and our ways of life. Because of this, we must be deliberate and prioritize the movements we were designed to make; we need to be intentional and ensure we take time to move often throughout the day. This is the best way to ask our brain to allow us to keep our strength and resiliency throughout our lives.

Pressing RESET daily will not only establish and improve the neural connections in our brain, but it will also establish our reflexive foundation of strength. The more we engage in The Big 5 RESETS, the deeper and more rooted our foundation becomes. Eventually, we will have a solid foundation strong enough to support any structure or lifestyle we want to create. This is the same process through which we built our original strength as a child. We showed up every day and lived in our design. We participated in creating our brains, and we strengthened our bodies through movement.

This is why Pressing RESET every day is so important. It grants us access to the bodies and, ultimately, the lives we want to have. It shapes our brains. It preserves our bodies. This is all made possible because the brain is plastic, it is always changing. Again, this is called neuroplasticity, and it is amazing! Think about it. Every thought and every movement you make alters the structure of your brain in some way by creating a new neural connection.[49]

The more you repeat a new thought or new movement, the more you etch that new neural connection into your brain. So, the more time you spend Pressing RESET, the more you engrave your foundational patterns and reestablish your original strength. As you engrave these connections, it becomes impossible to lose them as long as you keep using them.

Reestablishing your original strength is simply a matter of consistency. It is a simple addition. The more you show up and move, the more repetitions of movement you accumulate in your brain. The consistent addition of this accumulation of movement is a matter of choice. Whatever you do or do not do is born of choice. Whatever you choose is a positive or "negative" addition (subtraction). In other words, your choices add up in one direction or another; the direction you want to go or the direction you don't want to go.

If it is important for you to reestablish your original strength, you should choose to Press RESET every single day. By doing so, you leverage the math you need to restore your foundation and become as strong as you dream to be.

World-famous author and coach Dan John is often found quoting his mentor, Dan Gable, Olympic Gold Medalist and USA Wrestling Hall of Fame Member, with this phrase:

"If it is important, do it every day."

This is important. Press RESET every single day of your life. It is, after all, what you were designed to do...

The Ten-Minute Daily RESET

To get you started, here is a simple 10-minute daily RESET routine. It is almost too simple not to do. If you do this every day, it will make a difference in how you move and feel. This is a step towards restoring your original strength in mind and body. You can do this, and you should, every single day.

- Crocodile Breathe x 2 minutes.
  - o Keep your tongue on the roof of your mouth and breathe through your nose.
- Neck Nods from your hands and knees x 1 minute
- Segmental roll x 2 minutes.
  - o Perform segmental rolls from each limb.
  - o Remember to use your head when performing the upper body rolls!
- Rocking x 2 minutes.
  - o Explore rocking in plantar flexion (shoe laces down!) for 1 minute.
  - o Explore rocking in dorsiflexion (on the balls of your feet) for 1 minute.

- Hands and Knees Crawl x 2 minutes.
  - Keep your tongue on the roof of your mouth.
  - Keep your head up!
- Standing Cross-Crawls x 1 minute.

Warming Up

The above ten-minute daily reset can also be used as a warm-up before you engage in rigorous physical activity. These RESETS can make you "reflexively sharp" and enable you to express more of your strength and movement potential while reducing your chance of injury.

Speaking of warming up, have you ever seen a child stop and stretch or do jumping jacks before they run out on a playground? Nope. You've probably never seen that. No kid says, "Hey, wait and let me stretch," before they play a game of hide-n-seek. Kids don't need to warm up because they have their original strength or have a great deal of it.

If you begin Pressing RESET often and restore the foundation of your original strength, there may come a day when you do not have to stop and "warm up." You can regain the resiliency and readiness to play you had when you were a kid. It is all about resetting and restoring through repetition and the neurology of numerics. If you perform RESETS daily, you can eventually create a tipping point where your body is always ready for action. If your body is always ready for action, you do not need to warm up or prepare for action!

Now I know what I just said, but until that day comes, before you go out and play hide-n-seek, you should probably warm up by Pressing RESET for at least 10 minutes. Or at least play your first 10 minutes by walking instead of running.

Cooling Down

It is a good idea to gently move the body and work out any accumulated stress after rigorous physical activity. This can be known as cooling down. In swimming, this is called a "warm down." The above 10-minute daily reset can also make a wonderful cool down or warm down, depending on your terms.

Why?

Demanding physical activity, whether it be from heavy weight training, intense manual labor, or feats of physical endurance, can take a huge toll on the nervous system, fatiguing it. Demanding physical activity also requires a period of recovery. Pressing RESET after your body has been "through the ringer" is a great way to refresh your nervous system and minimize your recovery time.

Pressing RESET after physical exertion is another way to add repetition to your "RESET accumulation," deepening the roots of your original strength and getting you to the point where you are, once again, always ready for action because you are living in your design.

Restoring Life

"I'm an acupuncturist by day, a kettlebell instructor by night, and OS'er at all times. Anyway, this lady came to me in the clinic. Patient was an 80-year-old lady with major balance issues, having started five years ago but becoming quite severe over the last 2 to 3 years. During that time she had seen several MDs, one ENT and two neurologists.

Tests included but were not limited to CTs, an MRI, and a neural conduction test. All test results were unremarkable. Patient had suffered from numerous falls, which occurred without notice and in any direction. She was also unable to stand unsupported. Based on her history, I was able to rule out vertigo and lightheadedness. This seems like a reflexive stability issue.

The prescription... Neck nods, rocking, rolls, bird dogs, and seated marching. That was two weeks ago. I saw her for a follow-up today. After a couple of days of performing these exercises 3 to 4 times per day, she has had no further incidence of loss of balance. She is now walking easily, standing without support, and has even said goodbye to the upper and lower back pain that she used to have.

OS has not only given back this lady's quality of life but has probably also saved her life, considering her history of falls. On behalf of Mildred (who said to share her story freely), thank you to OS and all those who pioneered and advanced this incredible system."

—Daniel Hanscom
Canada

WHAT ABOUT STRETCHING AND MOBILITY WORK?

You probably don't need it.

This may be difficult for some of you, especially if you've been taught you need to stretch to be flexible and mobile.

Remember, the brain is always asking the question, "Am I safe?" Most of the time, if we are not living in our design, the answer to that question is "No."

If the answer is "No," the brain inhibits the body through various means, including tightness and immobility. I'm trying to say that being tight and immobile is often a safety mechanism placed on the body by the brain. If this is the case, performing stretching and mobility exercises would be an attempt to override the brain's safety protocols. I'm not sure that this is the best approach. It could even lead to an injury if the brain has a legitimate concern. And I can tell you, if you are not breathing in your design, the brain's concerns are legitimate.

You also probably know that stretching and mobility work doesn't work anyway, but you ignore that fact.

What are you talking about, Tim?

If stretching and mobility work *worked,* you wouldn't have to keep doing it over and over again. Or, to say it another way, if they worked, you wouldn't still be tight and immobile every single day. Stretching and mobility work are more of a ritual than an effective training modality. At best, they address the symptoms of inflexibility and immobility. Still, they do not address the roots of inflexibility and immobility.

Inflexibility and immobility are in your body to protect you from moving into dangerous situations. They are safeguards placed on your body by your brain because your brain has determined that something about you or something about what you are doing is not safe. To get to the root of this safety issue, you need to ensure that you are living and moving in your design.

When we live in our design, we restore our reflexive stability and mobility. I mentioned this earlier, but this is our reflexive strength. When we have our reflexive strength, we are MOBILE, FLEXIBLE, and STRONG. We don't need to stretch or perform myofascial release techniques because everything in us moves well.

Unless your sport is ballet or martial arts, or unless you are trying out for the next Gumby movie, you likely have all the flexibility and mobility you need **IF** you are Pressing RESET and living in your design. If you are in a specialized sport or need to be "super flexible," then yes, you may benefit from extra stretching. However, you should still stack that stretching on top of Pressing RESET.

But wait, if stretching and mobility work are more ritual than effective, why is Pressing RESET not a ritual? Don't we need to do that every day?

Yes and no.

You are designed to Press RESET every day. Every breath you take has the potential to let your brain know that you are safe. Every step you take should be restoring your nervous system. (This makes you want to listen to a certain song by the Police, doesn't it?) If we live in our design, we are constantly Pressing RESET. Until that happens, we need to Press RESET daily and often to tip the scales so that every breath, nod, and step is a RESET. This means Pressing RESET eventually gets to the point where it "sticks and stays."

Stretching and mobility work don't "stick and stay," even in the face of the SAID Principle, because they do not get to the root of the problem. The message of "I am not safe" is always being spoken, so the safety mechanisms of tightness and immobility are always reestablished. This is actually the SAID Principle, adapting the body to the "I am not safe" message. Do you see it?

This is to say that you probably don't need to stretch and perform mobility work. If you love the ritual and it makes you feel good, sure, do it. Just know that it is probably not doing what you think it is doing, and it just may be doing something you do not want it to do.

If you do stretch, you are probably better off not stretching before you engage in heavy weight training. Again, the safety mechanism of being tight may be protective for you.

When in doubt, before you train or embark on something physically strenuous, Press RESET. Let your brain know where everything is, and tell your brain you are safe. This will give you your best chance to move optimally and improve your performance.

You Must Become Converted Like a Child

Most health-related issues adults face can be traced to our modern-day lifestyle. In fact, according to a study in the *Annals of Internal Medicine*, which analyzed 47 different studies, too much sitting leads to early death due to the onset of chronic diseases like

Type 2 Diabetes, cardiovascular disease, and cancer.[50] If you have a creation that is made to move, a creation whose entire design is such that movement keeps it healthy. Confining it to an existence of not moving may be the fastest way to erode its health. Combine a sedentary lifestyle with a modern diet of new and foreign foods, and you can create a perfect storm of chronic disease.

But the answers to health and strength have always been hiding in plain sight, right before our eyes. Children live out these secrets every day. And if we pay attention to them and observe their ways, we can put their secrets to use. For example, have you ever noticed the peaceful and joyous expression on a child's face? They haven't been taught fear. They are living in a place of safety and joy. It's on their face, and when you see it, it actually makes you feel better. Their peace and joy are comforting to us. What if we also tried to live from a place of peace and safety? Or what if we at least breathed in such a way that our brain interpreted that we were safe?

But even consider what children do. Have you ever noticed how much a child will fight to stay out of a chair? Children have to be taught, nearly forced, to sit in chairs for anything longer than 2 minutes. At first, the chairs even have restraining bars to keep the child from escaping! We use the highchair, or the "safety seat," to keep the child seated and restrained. This violates the child's desire to move and explore his world. Yes, a highchair helps us attempt to enjoy our meals while it contains and restrains our children, but notice the battle that often ensues. Children are movers. Their bodies just *know* that they don't belong in chairs. It goes against their nature! They want to move, to live.

The child is the teacher. We should learn from them if we, too, want to be able to move and live. Consider the chair again. What do growing children do with chairs? They play with them. They turn chairs into a climbing gym, a monkey bar set, or a mountain that must be scaled and conquered. Not only do they grow and build their imaginations through learning how to move around a chair, but they also build their reflexive strength and enhance their nervous systems as they do so. When my children were 11 and 12 years old, they treated the chairs and couches in our house like parkour obstacles. They sucked me into doing the same. It was a lot of fun. Naturally, we only did this when my wife wasn't home.

The point is that we would be well suited to return to the simple ways of a child: move a lot, play, imagine, create, rest well, and eat well. This isn't as difficult as you might think. Your nature is to move............ We also need to learn from and listen to our own bodies. Your body knows it was made to move, and it tells you this every day. For example, how do you feel when you get out of a car after a 3 to 4-hour drive? Do you feel like you could run down a gazelle? Or do you feel like you are stiff and "old." Why do you feel so horrible? Because you haven't been moving!

Here is another way our bodies tell us about the importance of moving: Not moving ushers in boredom. Boredom is the death of your imagination. It is our imagination that keeps our brains healthy and ultimately keeps our bodies strong. The strength and health of a child and an adult are born out of imagination. You know this is true. Imagination gives birth to physical strength; "I wonder if I can climb that tree...", "That shiny, red ball sure does look awesome. I must get across the room to have it..."

When we are idle, the brain grows weary, tired, restless, and ultimately bored. Boredom leads to apathy, which is dangerous from a neurological perspective. If we practice not moving, we practice boredom and apathy. We become very good at these things in such a way that we are no longer good at moving, being creative, having vision, or having passion. Again, this leads to death or simply existing but not *living*.

> *"Where there is no vision, the people perish."*
> *—Proverbs 29:18*

The Power of Play

Every bit of a child's strength is developed through play and exploration. They do not "exercise." Exercise is a man-made concept adults created to develop strength and stamina. At best, exercise is a bandaid that tries to address the symptoms of not moving and living in our design. But children that grow up in play don't need to exercise. A creative, playful child becomes ounce for ounce stronger than most adults simply through learning how to move and engaging in play.

In the absence of play, I guess exercise makes some sense. But exercise is still work; it's not play. It can be boring, it can have too many rules, and it can be misapplied. That, along with the results of exercise, is fairly limited. For instance, adults can exercise to become strong and never come close to the strength and resiliency of a child.

Yes, adults can get stronger in the weight room, but they can't take a bench press outside of a gym. The ability to bench press a lot of weight will never *really* help you out in the world unless looking big-chested is helpful. But the bench press certainly won't help you go for a hike on a beautiful mountainside. Yet your ability to crawl, climb, play, and explore may give you everything you need to continue to live and enjoy life when you pass 90 years of age. In fact, living in your design will give you access to the natural and very powerful strength you already have tucked away inside your body. Pressing RESET removes inhibitions and limitations from the body, allowing you to perform optimally.

Children have more access to their natural strength and resiliency because they live to play and move, not exercise. This access is granted in stages. Once a child builds his foundation of reflexive strength by moving through his design and learning to crawl, walk, and run, he adds more strength and structure through exploration and play.

All the reflexive connections the child establishes along the way to walking get reinforced and sharpened as they explore their world through movement and play. The more they move and play, the more access they gain to their natural strength. Then, the more the child plays and challenges his body, the more strength and resiliency he builds. Again, this is all gradually done through a combination of curiosity, play, movement, and whimsical exploration—it's done through fun! And quite a bit of joy...

> **Adults attempt to use exercise in the same way a child uses play, except adults often leave out the "fun" part.**

It is the SAID Principle in action. Through play, a child learns how to challenge his body, and it is through consistent play that a child becomes successful at overcoming these challenges. This is the essence of strength; it is granted and built through adaptation.

Adults attempt to use exercise in the same way a child uses play, except adults often leave out the "fun" part. Through sets and reps, adults challenge their bodies and attempt to overcome the challenges in order to birth more strength. This does work for some, if it can be done consistently. However, for the majority of the population, exercise is not done consistently, if at all. For those who do attempt to exercise, many are often met with one failed attempt after another. What if they only fail because exercise isn't natural and doesn't leave them laughing, giggling and joyous?

Children often fail at play but don't care because they are having fun. A child can't instantly climb on monkey bars just because they are children. They have to build the strength it takes to climb the monkey bars through attempt after attempt, day after day. Can you see how a child intuitively masters the art of strength progression?

Adults cannot seem to do this. An adult wants to instantly be strong after one trip to the gym, or they want to instantly lose

30 pounds after one week of watching what they eat. Because of this mindset and the work it takes to succeed, most adults fail at building the health they want. Then, after they fail, they settle on the notion that they are just aging and "that's the way life is." This false notion has stolen many would-be amazing and adventurous lives. It leads to death (existence without real substance).

Please understand that I am not against exercise, nor am I saying that exercise leads to death. For some people, exercise actually is play; they love to exercise. Play can be anything you enjoy doing. It can be a game of basketball, riding a bike, going out for a run, climbing a tree, or even bench pressing and deadlifting. Play is anything that gets you moving and enjoying what you are doing while at the same time sparking your imagination or curiosity. The more fun it is, the better.

Have you ever noticed how hard it is to grow tired from play? Play begs you to keep going. It makes it easy for you to discover your strength. Exercise without play is just work. And when we have to work, we often tire pretty quickly.

Want to Play a Game?

Play has other benefits besides building health and strength. It nourishes the brain, establishing neural connections that enable the whole body to move better. It also helps relieve stress, improves energy, releases joy, improves creativity (builds up your imagination), and creates strong relationships between people.

Learning how to play brings people together and allows them to develop friendships and community. There is no better relationship builder between people. Play creates friends among acquaintances. Through games, play also teaches cooperation and teamwork, two of the most valuable skills a person can have. Playing games can actually develop teamwork in such a way that it might save your life.

Many moons ago, I was a firefighter stationed with eight other firefighters. Every morning, while we were on shift, we were required to participate in physical training for an hour. No one really enjoyed this but me. Training had been something I did and enjoyed from the time I was 13 years old.

Anyway, we were getting paid to exercise while at work, but there was no joy to be had in this "paid-to-exercise" time. Some firefighters would walk because that was the easiest thing to do in order to look like they were participating. Others would sit around on a weight bench or leisurely ride on a stationary bike. There was movement to satisfy the superiors, but no real training or exercise took place. Also, the firefighters at my station seemed to all be pretty "blah" or "just there." They never seemed too happy. There was no joy, and there was no camaraderie.

Note this: There was no camaraderie among men who would go into burning buildings together.

It was a job. We fought fires and answered EMS calls, not really in that order. And while we were on shift, we did our best to survive our time and stay out of trouble. We were just existing at work, on the job.

One day, we decided to shake things up and go to the local YMCA for our hour of physical training. If we left the station, there were supervising eyes on us. Somehow, while we were at the YMCA, a basketball game broke out. Naturally, this was against the rules of the department. We were supposed to exercise but not play sports. Sports were dangerous. That day, we were living on the edge! Do you know what happened next? Joy, hysterical laughter, and fun. Guys who typically never smiled nor got along started having fun together. We didn't want to leave. We could have played for hours.

Soon, every day when we came to work, we would drive the fire trucks to a field to play ultimate Frisbee or touch football. We started getting along and enjoying each other. The atmosphere at the fire station also changed. We were happy, and we liked each other. Being at work became enjoyable.

I can tell you that going into a burning building with people you care about and with people who care about you is a lot more comforting than going into a fire with people only there because it's their "job." In my fire station, playing games gave birth to friendship and teamwork. We built camaraderie.

Then someone got hurt, and we were told to quit playing games... But for a while, work was a blast!

The message here is that playing games with others can be a powerful RESET. It can even restore community. Don't dismiss this. We were made for community. Therefore, we need it.

As I just said, playing games also creates joy and laughter. Have you ever heard the saying, "A merry heart does good, like medicine?" This is true. Joy, fun, and laughter will keep you young. Joy is a RESEST in itself. It keeps sickness and depression at bay. And remember, joy is woven along with your movements. Being a kid at heart and engaging in play is a fantastic way to release your joy and free your body from limitations.

Ponder with me. What would happen if, a couple of times a week, you and your neighbors could get together and play hide-n-seek? I know what would happen. You would have fun and giggle your butt off. You would end up moving your body in all sorts of ways that you would never do being an "adult." Along with that, get your heart pumping, improve your cardiovascular system, and burn a ton of calories. You would also improve your coordination and spark creativity. Playing hide-n-seek with your neighbors would nourish your brain and strengthen your body. You would feel fantastic—*you would feel ALIVE!* You would be overcome with joy. How awesome would that be?

Can you imagine how good you would feel if you played a good game of hide-n-seek once or twice a week? Can you imagine the relationships you would build with your neighbors and the friendships you would grow? Could you do it? Could you love your neighbor as yourself? Yes, it is silly. But that doesn't make it wrong. Don't be afraid to act like a child. Learn to live. I'm not just telling this to you. I'm reminding myself as well. We all need more play and joy in our lives; we were meant to feel amazing.

Even if you don't fancy the idea of hide-n-seek with your neighbors, learn to use your imagination and find a way to play. Create your own games. They can be anything; it doesn't really matter what you choose to do. What matters is that you flex your "imagination muscle," have fun, and make play a regular part of your life.

Learning How to Play

Learning to play may feel weird initially, especially if your "imagination muscle" has atrophied. But remember, play can be anything. Most importantly, it gets you moving, and you enjoy it. You have the freedom to be creative and design your own play sessions. You can use your own creativity and do whatever you like. If you are really de-conditioned, start out gradually. Maybe set aside just ten minutes to go outside and play a few times a week. Learn to bounce a ball or practice your layups. As you start feeling better and more conditioned, increase your time and/or your level of activity. The bottom line is to do something on purpose to move and have fun. The more you do, the more you'll enjoy it.

If having the freedom to explore the idea of playing on your own seems stressful, it need not be. You cannot do this wrong as long as you do something. Play really can be anything that captures your imagination. Here are some examples:

1. Play dodgeball with your kids.
2. Go for a walk or a run in a park without your phone.

3. Go bike riding with some friends. Wear your helmet!
4. Play Pickleball! That is SO much fun.
5. Learn how to run sprints. Learn to skip first.
6. Climb a tree or play on some monkey bars. *Maybe wear a helmet.*
7. Learn to swim.
8. Play Frisbee golf.
9. Learn how to walk on a slack-line.
10. Learn how to tumble and take a fall.
11. Take Parkour lessons.
12. Play Hide-N-Seek!

If you engage in play, you'll find that your imagination and curiosity will grow. You may even discover that you enjoy challenging yourself with your preferred style of play. Eventually, you may find yourself doing things you never thought you would do, like signing up for a 5k or joining group bicycle rides. Curiosity may beg you to learn new skills and build new levels of physical strength simply because you start thinking things like, "I wonder if I can climb that tree?", "I wonder if I can hike all the way up that mountain?" If you build your "I wonder" muscles up, you will unlock new levels of strength and abilities you once dreamed of as a child. Learning to play is a great way to restore and retain your original strength. It keeps you young and vibrant and helps you see the world through a child's eyes.

Your parents meant well. When they told you to act your age, they probably didn't know they were stifling your growth and expression. We are meant to be young and wild at heart throughout life. Don't let the norms of society steal your youth. Being an adult doesn't have to mean you should put away fun, games, and joy. It doesn't mean you should resign your body from sports and fun activities and enlist only in the real world of work. Being an adult also doesn't mean it is okay to sit all day and stare at screens, intent on robbing your creativity and imagination.

Learn to play.

A Simple RESET Play Routine

If the previous examples of play are too extreme for you, try this:

Set aside 10 minutes three times a week to "play" by Pressing RESET. Learn to move in and out of the RESETS as you get up and down from the floor. Learn how to sit in all kinds of positions. Learn to go from crawling to sitting, from sitting to crawling to standing. Learn how to flow from one to the other. This is how you develop movement options. The more options you have, the better off you are. Options build resilience.

This is such a valuable time investment. How seamlessly can you flow in and out from rolling to crawling to kneeling to standing? How many different ways can you do this? How many different ways can you learn to stand without using your hands? Just play and explore! Use your imagination. Design strategies and techniques to move and get up from the ground. Build and learn options. When you can flow from one position to another, from the ground to standing and back down with grace, congratulations! You are stronger and more capable than you were when you started! This is a great way to add quality years of life to your body through play and exploration.

I Learned How to Play Again

"I visited the OS site and filled out the form to get the free guide to pressing reset. I was EXTREMELY skeptical at first because of how overhyped the movements seemed, but I tried it. I pressed reset with the Big 5, and I'm absolutely sure that it looked like a complete train wreck of an accident. I lifted my feet when I baby crawled and was probably hunched over. I couldn't even move in a contra-lateral pattern without having to think about it. Despite all that, after only a few minutes of moving, I stood up and instantly felt more free. I wanted to play with Karate again! I started punching and kicking and enjoying movement again right away. WOW! There was an INSTANT change in my body. It worked like a miracle. I knew from that point that this would be something that I'd do for the rest of my life.

Fast forward about 2 and a half years to the present. I feel AMAZING! Most importantly, I've learned to play again. I feel like I never got to play like I was supposed to when I was a kid, and learning how to play as an adult has been incredibly freeing. I still take things too seriously sometimes, but when I do, I play. I've learned how to find more balance in life. I can move in ways I couldn't before. I can kick and do Karate techniques in ways I couldn't before, even though I play with Karate very infrequently. I can skip, sprint, do front rolls, and do all sorts of stuff I had trouble doing well in the past. I can play with kettlebells without hurting my body now, too!

Most most importantly, I can play with my 5-year-old daughter and have a BLAST! We pretend to be Super Hero's almost every day, and my childhood has gone full circle and connected with hers in a healthy way that I never thought possible. I get to pretend I'm Leonardo, and she pretends that she's April, and we fight off the Foot Clan together. We play pretty hard every day, and right now, it's the primary form of my "training."

−Rick Evans
Arizona

THE MESSAGE OF STRENGTH

Ok, I know you're not going to play hide-n-seek with your neighbors. But you can build amazing strength by learning to play with your imagination and movements. This idea may be a little unnerving to some. If this is you, relax. You can always build strength through a more "mature," traditional approach. Regardless of how you desire to build strength, it is essential that you *do* build strength (on top of a solid foundation of reflexive strength, mobility, and stability), especially as you age. Strength enables you to live the life you were designed for.

This is the message: Strength enables you.

It gives you the capability of doing whatever it is you want to do. It makes whatever it is you are doing easier and better.

Life has challenges. There are physical tasks we need to be able to perform on a day-to-day basis to be successful. Every day you are able to take care of yourself, and those around you is a day of success. In light of this notion of success, failure is not an option.

Why do I equate having strength with being successful?

Because there will be a day, if it hasn't already come, when you value the strength needed to pick up and hold your own children, when you value the strength required to climb up and down your own stairs, or when you value the strength needed to put on your own shoes. Strength allows us to experience the simple victories of life, which most of us take for granted.

The truth is, most of us take strength for granted until we don't have it. When you don't have strength, you realize how vital it is for success in life. Without strength, joy, happiness, mental soundness, peace, freedom, and confidence all fade away. They fade away because if strength is the quality that enables you, weakness is the quality that incapacitates you. Being disabled through weakness brings depression, anxiety, mental turmoil, worry, fear, and doubt.

You need to be strong because strength makes life better.

A Simple Non-Traditional Strength Training Routine for Anyone

The following is a simple routine for those who want a little structure and guidance in building strength while not adhering to the traditional strength training model. This is a straightforward routine you can do almost anywhere. All you need is your body, a challenging object of mass, and two days a week to train (or two days a week to "play" for those who enjoy this).

First, pick two days a week to strength train, maybe Monday and Thursday or Tuesday and Saturday.

- Warm-up by Pressing RESET.
    - Crawl on your hands and knees for 10 minutes.
    - Hold your head up.
    - Keep your tongue on the roof of your mouth.
    - Breathe through your nose.
    - When your mouth pops open for air, rest!

- Let's go for 10 minutes of total work. If you have to rest, rest. But stop the clock. When you can continue on, start the clock.
- In time, the more capable you become, the less rest you need until you simply don't need to rest. This is AWESOME!
- Next, grab a challenging object of mass (a rock, a keg, a heavy dumbbell, any object…) and go for a 10 minute walk.

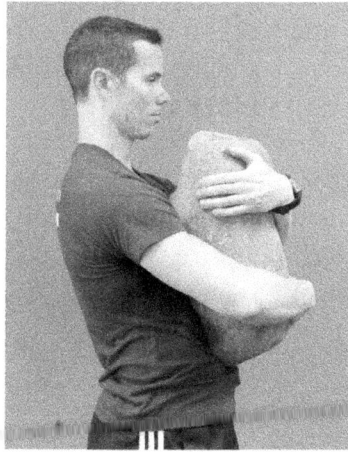

- Pick up an object and hold it in front of you if its shape allows.
- Walk about 10 yards and put the object down.
- Turn around, pick it up, and return to where you started.
- Repeat this over and over for 10 minutes.
- Keep your tongue on the roof of your mouth and breathe through your nose.
- If your mouth pops open, rest!
- Let's strive for 10 minutes of work. If you rest, stop the clock.
- Press RESET to cool down.
- Finally, take a quick 10-minute walk and let those arms swing from your shoulders.

Once you can crawl on your hands and knees for 10 minutes of work while breathing through your nose, it is time to progress! Start crawling backward on your hands and knees for 10 minutes of work, following the same rules as above.

Once you can complete this, progress to Leopard Crawling for 10 minutes of work, following the same rules.

Likewise, when you can carry your object of mass for 10 minutes of work, find a more challenging object to carry. It can be a bigger size, a different shape, or a heavier weight. A new challenge is a new opportunity to build more strength.

This simple strength training routine will surely enable you to become bulletproof in mind and body. Do not confuse simple with easy, however. This can be quite the challenge, and it is scalable to meet your abilities, whatever they are.

Simple, But So Effective

"After overtraining, my body was plagued by overuse injuries. Other than light kettlebell swings, the only other activity I could participate in comfortably was restorative yoga! I was desperate to return to the gym, but I had to find a way to train that would allow my body to heal rather than cause further injury. I immediately thought of Original Strength, so I signed up for their workshop and then followed that up by asking Tim to program my training sessions for a while!

The results of my training for the past year have been nothing short of phenomenal! I could not be happier! Not only did my previous injuries heal rather quickly while I trained using OS RESETS, crawling, and carries, but I rapidly grew much stronger! My body began working as a solid unit, and the strength skills I'd struggled with for years suddenly became easy.

For example, I was challenged to do Turkish Get Ups for reps using a 12kg kettlebell a year ago. Fast forward a year, and I'm able to do Turkish Get Ups with an 18kg KB…and for multiple reps! I used to dread doing single-leg deadlifts as I was wobbly using even the 4kg kettlebell. Now I'm doing sets of 5/5 using a 20kg kettlebell!

I could go on and on about all the cool strength skills that have improved significantly after primarily crawling and carrying for the past year. But the most incredible effect of incorporating Pressing RESET into my training program is how efficiently and gracefully my body now moves!

At the age of 56, I'm still amazed, daily, how effortlessly I'm able to move about and perform daily activities that at one time were painful! If performing OS RESETS keeps my body youthful, count me in…I will be rocking, rolling, and crawling well into my 90s!"

–Patricia Olsen
Nashville

Traditional Training Templates

For those of you who are "in the box" thinkers!

The following templates are for those of you who desire a more traditional, more structured strength training approach using weights. Simply use these templates with your current weight training program. It is easy to integrate the principles of Original Strength into any training regimen.

Note: I'm going to provide some examples of what a week's training program may look like for each week scenario below. I'm warning you because I'm also going to weave some creativity into these examples. So, if you are an "in the box" thinker, practice your nasal breathing while you look at my examples. It's going to be ok!

<u>3 Days A Week</u>

> Day 1: Press RESET, Barbell Strength Work*, Conditioning, Press RESET
>
> Day 2: Press RESET, Barbell Strength Work*, Conditioning, Press RESET
>
> Day 3: Press RESET, Barbell Strength Work*, Conditioning, Press RESET

*Substitute Barbell Strength Work with Kettlebells, Dumbbells, Bodyweight, or whatever you fancy.

Here is an example of what this might look like:

Day 1 (Monday):

Press RESET x 10 min:

- Breathe x 2 min
- Head Nods and Rotations x 2 min

- Rolling x 2 min
- Rocking x 2 min
- Cross-Crawls x 2 min

Barbell Strength Work:

- Deadlifts x 5 sets of 3
- Military Press x 5 sets of 5

Conditioning:

- Farmers Carries with bodyweight x 10 minutes of work

Press RESET x 5 minutes

- Segmental Rolling for 5 minutes

Day 2 (Wednesday):

Press RESET x 10 min:

- Breathe x 2 min
- Head Nods and Rotations x 2 min
- Rolling x 2 min
- Rocking x 2 min
- Cross-Crawls x 2 min

Barbell Strength Work:

- Bench Press x 5 sets of 5
- Triceps Extensions x 3 sets of 10
- Chin-ups x 4 sets of 8
- Biceps Curls x 3 sets of 10

Conditioning:

- Leopard Crawling x 10 minutes of work

Press RESET x 5 minutes

- Crocodile Breathing x 5 minutes

Day 3 (Friday):

Press RESET x 10 min:

- Breathe x 2 min
- Head Nods and Rotations x 2 min
- Rolling x 2 min
- Rocking x 2 min
- Cross-Crawls x 2 min

Barbell Strength Work:

- Back Squats x 5 sets of 5
- Bent Over Rows x 5 sets of 5

Conditioning:

- Single-arm Overhead Carries with 20-30% bodyweight x 10 minutes of work

Press RESET x 5 minutes

- Rocking x 5 minutes

4 Days A Week

> Day 1: Press RESET, Barbell Strength Work, Conditioning, Press RESET
>
> Day 2: Press RESET, Kettlebell Strength Work, Conditioning, Press RESET
>
> Day 3: Press RESET, Kettlebell Strength Work, Conditioning, Press RESET
>
> Day 4: Press RESET, Barbell Strength Work, Conditioning, Press RESET

Here is an example of what this might look like:

Day 1 (Monday):

Press RESET x 10 min:

- Breathe x 2 min
- Head Nods and Rotations x 2 min
- Rolling x 2 min
- Rocking x 2 min
- Cross-Crawls x 2 min

Barbell Strength Work:

- Deadlifts x 5 sets of 3
- Military Press x 5 sets of 5

Conditioning:

- Single-arm Suitcase Carries with 30% bodyweight x 10 minutes of work

Press RESET x 5 minutes

- Segmental Rolling for 5 minutes

Day 2 (Tuesday):

Press RESET x 10 min:

- Breathe x 2 min
- Head Nods and Rotations x 2 min
- Rolling x 2 min
- Rocking x 2 min
- Cross-Crawls x 2 min

Kettlebell Strength Work:

- Turkish Getups x 5 sets of 5r/5l
- Goblet Squats x 3 sets of 10

Conditioning:

- Leopard Crawling x 10 minutes of work

Press RESET x 10 minutes

- Brisk Walk with very light weighted backpack x 10 minutes

Day 3 (Thursday):

Press RESET x 10 min:

- Breathe x 2 min
- Head Nods and Rotations x 2 min
- Rolling x 2 min
- Rocking x 2 min
- Cross-Crawls x 2 min

Kettlebell Strength Work:

- Two-handed Swings x 10 sets of 10
- Push-press x 5 sets of 8r/8l

Conditioning:

- Farmers Carries with bodyweight x 10 minutes of work

Press RESET x 5 minutes

- Rocking x 5 minutes

Day 4 (Friday):

Press RESET x 10 min:

- Breathe x 2 min
- Head Nods and Rotations x 2 min
- Rolling x 2 min
- Rocking x 2 min
- Cross-Crawls x 2 min

Barbell Strength Work:

- Back Squats x 5 sets of 5
- Bent Over Rows x 5 sets of 5

Conditioning:

- Single-arm Overhead Carries with 20-30% bodyweight x 10 minutes of work

Press RESET x 10 minutes

- Brisk Walk with very light weighted backpack x 10 minutes

<u>5 Days A Week</u>

> Day 1: Press RESET, Strength Work, Press RESET
> Day 2: Press RESET, Conditioning, Press RESET
> Day 3: Press RESET, Strength Work, Press RESET
> Day 4: Press RESET, Conditioning, Press RESET
> Day 5: Press RESET, Strength Work, Press RESET

Here is an example of what this might look like:

Day 1 (Monday):

Press RESET x 10 min:

- Breathe x 2 min
- Head Nods and Rotations x 2 min
- Rolling x 2 min
- Rocking x 2 min
- Cross-Crawls x 2 min

Barbell Strength Work:

- Power Cleans x 5 sets of 3
- Push-Press x 5 sets of 5

Conditioning:

- Single-arm Suitcase Carries with 30% bodyweight x 10 minutes of work

Press RESET x 5 minutes

- Segmental Rolling for 5 minutes

Day 2 (Tuesday):

Press RESET x 10 min:

- Breathe x 2 min
- Head Nods and Rotations x 2 min
- Rolling x 2 min
- Rocking x 2 min
- Cross-Crawls x 2 min

Conditioning (Sprints):

- Leopard Crawl x 20 yards, walk back
- Cross-Crawl x 20 yards, walk back
- March x 20 yards, walk back
- Skip x 20 yards, walk back
- Bound x 20 yards, walk back
- Repeat all
- Sprint x 80 yards, walk back
    - Repeat for a total of 5 sprints

Press RESET

- Skip x 20 yards, walk back
- March x 20 yards, walk back
- Cross-Crawl x 20 yards, walk back
- Leopard Crawl x 20 yards, walk back

Day 3 (Wednesday):

Press RESET x 10 min:

- Breathe x 2 min
- Head Nods and Rotations x 2 min
- Rolling x 2 min
- Rocking x 2 min
- Cross-Crawls x 2 min

Kettlebell Strength Work:

- Rack Squats (moderate to light) x 3 sets of 5r/5l
- Kettlebell Snatches x 10 sets of 5r/5l

Conditioning <u>and</u> RESET:

- Brisk Ruck with light loaded backpack x 20 minutes

Day 4 (Thursday):

Press RESET x 10 min:

- Breathe x 2 min
- Head Nods and Rotations x 2 min
- Rolling x 2 min
- Rocking x 2 min
- Cross-Crawls x 2 min

Conditioning (Sprints):

- Leopard Crawl x 20 yards, walk back
- Cross-Crawl x 20 yards, walk back
- March x 20 yards, walk back
- Skip x 20 yards, walk back
- Bound x 20 yards, walk back
- Repeat all
- Sprint x 80 yards, walk back
    - Repeat for a total of 8 sprints

Press RESET

- Skip x 20 yards, walk back
- March x 20 yards, walk back
- Cross-Crawl x 20 yards, walk back
- Leopard Crawl x 20 yards, walk back

Day 5 (Friday):

Press RESET x 10 min:

- Breathe x 2 min
- Head Nods and Rotations x 2 min
- Rolling x 2 min
- Rocking x 2 min
- Cross-Crawls x 2 min

Barbell Strength Work:

- Front Squats x 5 sets of 5
- Pull-ups x 10 sets of 5

Conditioning:

- Single-arm Overhead Carries with 20-30% bodyweight x 10 minutes of work

Press RESET x 5 minutes

- Hands and Knees Crawling x 5 minutes

> Day 1: Press RESET, Strength Work, Press RESET
> Day 2: Press RESET, Conditioning, Press RESET
> Day 3: Press RESET, Strength Work, Press RESET
> Day 4: Press RESET, Conditioning, Press RESET
> Day 5: Press RESET, Strength Work, Press RESET
> Day 6: Press RESET, Conditioning, Press RESET

Here is an example of what this might look like:

Day 1 (Monday):

Press RESET x 10 min:

- Breathe x 2 min
- Head Nods and Rotations x 2 min
- Rolling x 2 min
- Rocking x 2 min
- Cross-Crawls x 2 min

Strength Work:

- Turkish Getup Practice x 10 minutes
- Two-handed Swings x 10 reps, as many rounds as possible for 10 minutes
- Chin-ups x 5 reps, as many rounds as possible for 10 minutes

Press RESET x 5 minutes

- Segmental Rolling for 5 minutes

Day 2 (Tuesday):

Press RESET x 10 min:

- Breathe x 2 min

- Head Nods and Rotations x 2 min
- Rolling x 2 min
- Rocking x 2 min
- Cross-Crawls x 2 min

Conditioning:

- Farmer's Carries and Backwards Leopard Crawls x 20 minutes
  - Farmer's Carry two bells 20 yards and put them down
  - Backwards Leopard Crawl for 30 steps. Stand up and walk back to the bells.
  - Repeat sequence for 20 minutes

Press RESET x 5 minutes

- Rocking x 5 minutes

Day 3 (Wednesday):

Press RESET x 10 min:

- Breathe x 2 min
- Head Nods and Rotations x 2 min
- Rolling x 2 min
- Rocking x 2 min
- Cross-Crawls x 2 min

Strength Work:

- Hindu Squats x 20 reps, as many rounds and possible for 10 minutes
- Pushups x 10 reps, as many rounds as possible for 10 minutes
- TRX Rows x 10 reps, as many rounds as possible for 10 minutes

Press RESET x 3 minutes

- Elevated Rolling for 3 minutes

Day 4 (Thursday):

Press RESET x 10 min:

- Breathe x 2 min
- Head Nods and Rotations x 2 min
- Rolling x 2 min
- Rocking x 2 min
- Cross-Crawls x 2 min

Strength Work:

- Turkish Getup Practice x 10 minutes
- Two-handed Swings x 10 reps, as many rounds as possible for 10 minutes
- Chin-ups x 5 reps, as many rounds as possible for 10 minutes

Press RESET x 5 minutes

- Segmental Rolling for 5 minutes

Day 5 (Friday):

Press RESET x 10 min:

- Breathe x 2 min
- Head Nods and Rotations x 2 min
- Rolling x 2 min
- Rocking x 2 min
- Cross-Crawls x 2 min

Conditioning:

- Farmer's Carries and Backwards Leopard Crawls x 20 minutes
  - Farmer's Carry two bells 20 yards and put them down
  - Backwards Leopard Crawl for 30 steps. Stand up and walk back to the bells.
  - Repeat sequence for 20 minutes

Press RESET x 5 minutes

- Rocking x 5 minutes

Day 6 (Saturday):

Press RESET x 10 min:

- Breathe x 2 min
- Head Nods and Rotations x 2 min
- Rolling x 2 min
- Rocking x 2 min
- Cross-Crawls x 2 min

Strength Work:

- Hindu Squats x 20 reps, as many rounds and possible for 10 minutes
- Pushups x 10 reps, as many rounds as possible for 10 minutes
- TRX Rows x 10 reps, as many rounds as possible for 10 minutes

Press RESET x 3 minutes

- Elevated Rolling for 3 minutes

Other Ideas

There is no one way to plan your training and over a million ways to skin a cat. Here are some other ideas of how a week of training could look:

3 Days A Week

Day 1: Barbell Strength Training
Day 2: Bodyweight Training
Day 3: Original Strength

    Sample:

    Monday: Military Press, Front Squat
    Wednesday: Chins, Parallel Dips, Hindu Squats
    Friday: Leopard Crawl for time

Day 1: Kettlebell Training
Day 2: Bodyweight Training
Day 3: Original Strength

    Sample:

    Monday: Get Ups, Swings, Presses
    Wednesday: Chins, Parallel Dips, Hindu Squats
    Friday: Leopard Crawls for time

4 Days A Week

Day 1: Barbell and Kettlebell
Day 2: Bodyweight and Original Strength
Day 3: Barbell and Kettlebell
Day 4: Bodyweight and Original Strength

Sample:

Monday: Military Press, Front Squat, Swings
Tuesday: Chins, Dips, Crawling
Thursday: Deadlift, Bench Press, Swings
Friday: Handstand Push ups, Hindu Squats, Crawling

5 Days A Week

Day 1: Barbell Training
Day 2: Original Strength
Day 3: Bodyweight Training
Day 4: Original Strength
Day 5: Kettlebell Training

Sample:

Monday: Deadlift, Military Press, Front Squat
Tuesday: Crawling
Wednesday: Chins, Handstand Push Ups, Hindu Squats
Thursday: Crawling
Friday: Get Ups, Swings, Goblet Squats

Reset Your Training

Besides Pressing RESET before and after you train, you can also Press RESET while you train.

In fact, Pressing RESET during your training sessions will make them more effective because it allows you to recover faster, even between sets.

For example, heavy weight training stresses the body. It taxes the nervous system and tires the muscles. It can even weigh on the mind. Once the body is stressed, performing consecutive sets with the same focus, energy, and strength that was applied to the first "heavy" set can be challenging. As the sets in a training session go on, the quality of the movements can degrade with each stressful, taxing repetition.

Pressing RESET in between your sets allows you to restore the body's nervous system to a relaxed and ready state, thus enabling you to perform well on your next set, from set to set. Instead of losing the quality of your movement and increasing your risk for injury, you improve your movements and reduce your chance of injury. That is the goal, right?

If you strength train, you should be training to get strong in a safe and effective manner. Your goal should be to have strength so you can enjoy your life and/or perform well at your sport. Even if you treat strength training as your sport, you probably agree that in order for you to be happy, you need to be able to train. So, it would only make sense that your strength training routine should be built around quality movements and not merely the quantity of movements.

Pressing RESET between your strength training sets can help you maintain quality movements throughout your entire training session. It *resets* you. It even improves your strength, speed, power, and focus while you train, allowing you to maintain quality of movement and thus lowering your chances of injury due to training.

Try this yourself. Take a weight that you struggle to press one to two times and press it. Then, get on the floor and rock back and forth ten times. Now press the weight again. You probably found that the weight went up easier, and/or you were able to press it more times than you did the first time. Pressing RESET works.

We are all a bit different. In your own training, you may find certain RESETS work very well when paired with certain exercises. For example, rocking in between sets of squats may really improve your squat session. Performing head nods between sets of overhead presses may give you more power to press. This is where the fun of RESET experimentation comes into play. Play—*there's that word again*. Playing with the RESETS inside of your training session is a great way to learn how your body responds to certain RESETS and how they improve your performance. This is how I learned how powerful Marching is as a reset. It made me stronger and better when I marched between my weight training sets.

If you're not into playing and exploring yet, just superset all your training sets with proper breathing. You can stand in the power pose with your hands around your waist (stand like Superman), close your lips, place your tongue on the roof of your mouth, and breathe in and out through your nose. Make sure you are getting air inside the bottom of your lungs. If this is all you did, you'd be Pressing RESET, and your training sets would be smooth, pretty, and strong. Breath is life; when we breathe in our design, everything works better.

Just remember, **there are no rules.** You can perform the RESET you feel you need. If you don't know what you need, breathe. But just in case, to give you some ideas, here are some examples of how this might look.

Movement RESETS

- Rocking x 10 reps, followed by 2 Hand Swings x 10 - 20 reps
- Goblet Squats x 5 reps, followed by Marching x 20 steps
- Back squats x 3 - 5 reps, followed by elevated rolls x 2 rolls with each leg
- Neck nods x 10 reps, followed by Clean and Press x 3 - 5 reps
- Strict overhead presses x 3 reps, followed by marching or cross-crawls x 20 steps
- Heavy Deadlifts x 1 - 3 reps, followed by elevated rocking x 10 reps
- Sprinting x 60 yards, followed by rocking x 20 reps
- Pull-ups x 5 - 10 reps, crocodile breathing x 5 slow breaths
- Leopard Crawling x 20 reps, followed by a barbell Clean & Jerk x 1 - 3 reps

Again, there are no rules here. Experiment with the RESETS and use the ones that tend to relax and restore you the most. You may be pleasantly surprised to find your movements get better and better as you train. You will also benefit from ending your training sessions feeling refreshed and invigorated. This should be the point; your training should build you up, not tear you down.

THE ORIGINAL NUTRITION STRATEGY

Regarding growing strong and healthy, nutrition matters - A LOT.

However, nutrition is a tricky subject to tackle, not because of its complexity but because of the belief systems and information that infiltrate nutrition. Nutrition is essential, if not paramount, to how well your body functions. The problem is there is SO much information, misinformation, and varying beliefs where "experts" completely disagree on what to eat when to eat, and even how to eat. Nutrition is like the Wild West; every expert has a duel at high noon to shoot the other down.

There is also the issue of our individuality; what my body thrives on may not be what your body thrives on. Anyway, the chaotic abyss of nutritional information can really drive a person crazy. The more you learn about nutrition, the more you can end up chasing your tail. And that can be very frustrating.

For example, in the first edition of this book, "Paleo" nutrition was popular: Low carb, natural whole foods, with an emphasis on meat and natural fats. It was supposed to be the "healthiest" way to live. And it may be, for some. Since that edition, Veganism, Vegan-Keto, Keto, Ketovore, and Carnivore have become popular.

It's kind of a lot. No matter your views or beliefs, I think everyone can agree that not eating ultra-processed foods is the way to go. Especially not eating ultra-processed carbohydrates.

Beyond that, different peoples and cultures should or would have different diets because they live in various geographical locations that produce different available foods depending on their climates, soils, and water supplies. To extrapolate one area's eating habits and blanket them on the whole of society may not be wise. Depending on our genetic inheritance, we likely have differences in the foods we can thrive with or the foods we can survive with.

For example, people of European descent seem to be able to digest milk and consume it without too many issues. But that is not the case for the rest of the world. Why should someone living in Alaska think the Mediterranean diet would be the best for them? They may not be the best application of information for their particular genetics and environment.

Also, consider that our world has seasons. People once ate what was available in their location in its season. Certain foods only grow at certain times of the year. Or at least that is how it would naturally be.

Now, with modern agricultural practices and technologies, there are no seasons. Your grocery store always has food, in and out of season. Seasons help cycle our foods and give us variety. Seasons also provide us with nutrition and flavor. Have you ever noticed how great strawberries taste in their season and how "blah" they taste in the winter? Seasons are seasons for a reason.

Having said all that, I'd like to share a few things about nutrition:

1. The body is made to thrive and not just survive. Yes, the body is excellent at adapting, but ideally, the body is made to thrive and flourish. Eating ultra-processed foods can put the body in "survival mode." The consequences of living

on ultra-processed foods are high. It can lead to disease and chronic illness. No matter how good movement is for us, it can't remove the poisons we willingly ingest.

2. We were made to move. And, we were made to eat. We have tastebuds for a reason. It is okay for food to taste good and be enjoyed. Also, if food tastes like "bleck" maybe it is okay not to eat it. Life is made to be lived, and therefore, food can be enjoyed. Just don't let food consume and imprison you.

3. Food is information. Information leads to our expression. If you want to feel your best, consume the best information. Your body knows what to do with real food. There is a chance it just does the best it can with Frankenfoods.

4. We were not made to eat preservatives, additives, artificial sweeteners, Red Dye #66, or any other "natural" flavor or *generally recognized as a safe or almost safe* chemical that you can think of. If the food you eat was designed by man to have a long shelf-life, then it will probably shorten your shelf-life. You do not have a food additive chemical deficiency! The closer your food is to the way God made it, the better off you probably are.

5. Eat what you are. I'll leave it at that.

At best, this section is really just "food for thought." If you read the first edition of this book, you can see my views on nutrition have shifted or even matured. That's because a young body can get away with more than a more mature body. The margin of error for the mature body is much smaller. Just know that to live your best life, nutrition is critical in regaining and keeping our original strength.

When in doubt, eat whole, natural food. Stop eating when you're full. Go outside and get some sun. Go for walks. Get a good night's sleep. These are all forms of nutrition.

MANAGE YOUR EXPECTATIONS

If you are reading this book, I imagine you are not satisfied with the thought of living with movement issues, injuries, age-related issues, weakness, fatigue, apathy, or any limitations. You want more for yourself than just sitting around and watching life go by. You want to have "Golden Years" and not tarnished brass years. In other words, you want to LIVE!

Here is a question for you: *What are you expecting?*

Are you expecting to be strong, healthy, and resilient? Do you believe you will regain your original strength? Or do you imagine yourself sick, weak, overweight, and lifeless? Another way to ask this is: What do you see when you "see" yourself in your mind's eye?

The answer(s) to these questions is extremely important. You will become the way you think and get what you expect. Likely, you do have what you've been expecting. Where the mind goes, the body will follow.

If you believe you can regain the body you were meant to have, you will. If you believe you will end up in a rest home, you probably will. The thoughts you keep in your head get planted in your heart, shaping your beliefs, which determines your outcome.

You might be thinking that I'm getting a little spiritual right now, you might be right. However, there is very much a physical truth to what I'm saying here. Truth always has parallels.

Every single action you make, every single thought you have, actually changes the structure of your brain in order for your brain to become more efficient.[51] The brain strives for efficiency. A neural connection is made when you have a thought, good or bad. This connection allows that thought to become more efficient. The more you think that same thought, the more you literally cement that thought into your brain.[52]

Yes, it is true: Eventually, it takes *less thought* to have that same thought! Remember, the brain operates on the "use it and keep it" principle. The more you entertain a thought, the more you cement the neural connection that was made by that thought, and the easier it is to have that thought. Your thoughts can become common to your brain. In other words, you can create *habitual* thoughts, good or bad. These habitual thoughts will eventually manifest in your body and in your life.

This is *one* reason why controlling your thoughts and imagination is imperative. When you see yourself in the future, you need to see yourself strong. You need to see yourself conquering mountains, climbing trees, sprinting down rabbits, or whatever boss-mode action you can think of. You need to believe and *know* you are capable and able to overcome obstacles. You need to see yourself ALIVE!

If you are injured now, you need to know that soon, you will be healed. "This too shall pass" - make that your mantra. Soon, you will be resilient. For instance, if you can't walk up a flight of stairs without gasping for air, you need to believe you'll be bounding up those same stairs with ease in just a few short weeks.

Put good, positive thoughts—the images you want to become, the things you want to do—inside your head and keep them there.

Think about them over and over. Those thoughts will create habitual thoughts and end up shaping your beliefs. You know this to be true. Think of someone who always worries or who is always negative. Are they fun to be around? No, probably not. How do those people act? Are they full of life and energy? No, probably not. Now, think about how those people move and look. Do they move with strength and grace? Is their posture perfect? Or do they slump? Is their head protruded forward?

Are their shoulders rounded forward as well? Yes, probably so.

Negative thoughts are "dead" thoughts. Dead things sink to the bottom of the lake, decompose, and waste away. Positive thoughts are "alive", they have life in them. Things that are alive rise to the top. They thrive.

Our thoughts present themselves in our bodies and our lives. We reflect how we think. If you want to be strong, if you want to have vitality, think strong! Think vitality, think LIFE! Remember, your thoughts actually change the physical shape of your brain. Thoughts become real, physical things! If you are going to change the shape of your brain, change it for the better. Expect health. Expect strength. Expect life!

And yes, this is also spiritual. Proverbs 23:7 says, *"For as he thinks in his heart, so is he."*

Simple wisdom makes for simple reality.

This may not be what you were expecting to find near the back of this book, but this could be the most important chapter of the whole book! If you want to regain your original strength, you must think and believe you will. It is that simple.

It's Amazing

"I used to have neck pain, spasms, tightness, limited range of motion on the left side of my neck and even headaches. I was going to acupuncture for it. Since doing daily OS RESETS since the workshop on January 11 I have had zero neck pain, stiffness or headaches. I have a new range of motion that I have never had before and I can now touch my chin to my chest. It's like I have a whole new neck haha! It's pretty amazing!"

—Artemis Scantalides
Massachusetts

THE END?

When I decided to write this book and present this information, I only wanted to share what I've learned and help people become as resilient as possible. This is important because a healthy, strong body paves the way to a healthy, happy life.

There is a lot of excellent training and movement information in the world. There are also many different schools of thought on the best ways to move to improve one's health. All of them have lots of great information to offer. None are complete, and many contradict each other. I'm not saying other movement and training systems or methodologies are "wrong" or that the information I'm presenting is "right" or better than anyone else's training system. But I will say that your Original Strength, the movement template you were born with, is THE foundation of everything else and all other methods and systems. Learning to Press RESET and living in your design will only improve your experience and expression in all other training systems and movement modalities.

> **I believe, and with good reason, that Original Strength is the foundation for life, health, and longevity.**

I believe, and with good reason, that Original Strength is the foundation for life, health, and longevity. It is the original default operating system, the foundation for anything you want to do or become. Living in your design allows you to live your life better.

Aside from that, I've had a childhood fantasy of being Superman for over 49 years. I want to be physically capable of saving the day, conquering obstacles, or being useful. I don't want to hurt, I don't want to struggle with fear, I don't want to know kryptonite. I used to think this was silly and that something was wrong with me until I read John Eldridge's book *Wild at Heart*.

I believe this idea was planted inside me before I was born, just like my movement operating system. Original Strength was an answer to my prayer to be like Superman. I know this answer was not just for me. We've all been given the same movement template, we were all meant to be strong, resilient, capable, and dependable. We were all meant to save the day and to be useful to those around us. This is truth.

Please put the information in this book to the test. Give yourself a few months and engage in the RESETS consistently. Expect good things to happen in your body and in your life. And be patient. Remember, Rome wasn't built in a day. But it was built. It took time and consistent effort to build one of the most amazing empires the world has ever known. So it is true with your body. **Regaining your Original Strength is a journey.** But it is a journey worth exploring. Give yourself time and enjoy the journey.

I'll end this as I started it: We are all, every single one of us, awesomely and wonderfully made. Keep this in your heart, and don't believe anything or anyone that suggests otherwise.

God Loves You.

ENDNOTES

1. United States Luge Association, "What Makes a Successful Luge Athlete?" www.teamusa.org/usa-luge/rules-and-policies, accessed July 1, 2015

2. American Physical Therapy Association, 2013 House of Delegates Minutes, www.apta.org/HOD/, accessed June 28, 2015.

3. Seidler RD. Neural Correlates of Motor Learning, Transfer of Learning, and Learning to Learn. Exercise and sport sciences reviews. 2010;38(1):3-9. doi:10.1097/JES.0b013e3181c5cce7.

4. Sally Goddard Blythe, The Well Balanced Child (Stroud: Hawthorne Press, 2005), p. xiv.

5. Carla Hannaford, Smart Moves (Salt Lake City: Great River Books, 2005), p. 48.

6. Carla Hannaford, Smart Moves (Salt Lake City: Great River Books, 2005), p. 32.

7. Carla Hannaford, Smart Moves (Salt Lake City: Great River Books, 2005), p. 28.

8. Sally Goddard Blythe, The Well Balanced Child (Stroud: Hawthorne Press, 2005), p. 176.

9. Sally Goddard Blythe, The Well Balanced Child (Stroud: Hawthorne Press, 2005), p. 23.

10. Barry Ross, Underground Secrets to Faster Running (BearPowered.com, 2005), p. 62.

11. Carla Hannaford, Smart Moves (Salt Lake City: Great River Books, 2005), p. 111.

12. https://www.sciencedaily.com/releases/2013/05/130501193204.htm

13. Sally Goddard Blythe, The Well Balanced Child (Stroud: Hawthorne Press, 2005), p. 35.

14. Carla Hannaford, Smart Moves (Salt Lake City: Great River Books, 2005), p. 39.

15. Idem.

16. Carla Hannaford, Smart Moves (Salt Lake City: Great River Books, 2005), p. 38.

17. Sally Goddard Blythe, The Well Balanced Child (Stroud: Hawthorne Press, 2005), p. 13.

18. Carla Hannaford, Smart Moves (Salt Lake City: Great River Books, 2005), p. 38.

19. Sally Goddard Blythe, Reflexes, Learning and Behavior (Eugene: Fern Ridge Press, 2005), p. 20.

20. Carla Hannaford, Smart Moves (Salt Lake City: Great River Books, 2005), p. 49.

21. Sally Goddard Blythe, Reflexes, Learning and Behavior (Eugene: Fern Ridge Press, 2005), p. 59.

22. Idem.

23. Carla Hannaford, Smart Moves (Salt Lake City: Great River Books, 2005), p. 39.

24. Sally Goddard Blythe, The Well Balanced Child (Stroud: Hawthorne Press, 2005), p. 18.

25. Sally Goddard Blythe, The Well Balanced Child (Stroud: Hawthorne Press, 2005), p. 19.

26. Idem.

27. Carla Hannaford, Smart Moves (Salt Lake City: Great River Books, 2005), p. 111.

28. Carla Hannaford, Smart Moves (Salt Lake City: Great River Books, 2005), p. 134.

29. http://www.theatlantic.com/health/archive/2014/11/what-texting-does-to-the-spine/382890/

30. Deane Juhan, Job's Body: A Handbook for Bodywork (Barrytown, NY: Station Hill Press, 2003), p. 24.

31. Ibid. p. 45.

32. Gray Cook, Movement (Santa Cruz: On Target Publications, 2010), pps. 187-189.

33. www.functionalmovement.com

34. Carla Hannaford, Smart Moves (Salt Lake City: Great River Books, 2005), p. 173.

35. Carla Hannaford, Smart Moves (Salt Lake City: Great River Books, 2005), p. 91.

36. Carla Hannaford, Smart Moves (Salt Lake City: Great River Books, 2005), p. 112.

37. Carla Hannaford, Smart Moves (Salt Lake City: Great River Books, 2005), p. 112.

38. Idem.

39. Sally Goddard Blythe, The Well Balanced Child (Stroud: Hawthorne Press, 2005), p. 185.

40. Idem.

41. Idem.

42. Idem.

43. http://www.cbsnews.com/news/living-to-90-and-beyond/

44. Pavel Tsatsouline, Power to the People (St. Paul: Dragon Door Publications, 1999), p. 78.

45. Pavel Tsatsouline, Power to the People (St. Paul: Dragon Door Publications, 1999), p. 79.

46. Norman Doidge, The Brain that Changes Itself (New York: The Penguin Group, 2007), p. 208.

47. http://en.wikipedia.org/wiki/SAID_principle

48. Sally Goddard Blythe, The Well Balanced Child (Stroud: Hawthorne Press, 2005), p. 23.

49. Norman Doidge, The Brain that Changes Itself (New York: The Penguin Group, 2007), p. 208.

50. "Sedentary Time and Its Association With Risk for Disease Incidence, Mortality, and Hospitalization in Adults: A Systematic Review and Meta-analysis." Aviroop Biswas, BSc; Paul I. Oh, MD, MSc; Guy E. Faulkner, PhD; Ravi R. Bajaj, MD; Michael A. Silver, BSc; Marc S. Mitchell, MSc; and David A. Alter, MD, PhD. Annals of Internal Medicine. January 20, 2015.

51. Norman Doidge, The Brain that Changes Itself (New York: The Penguin Group, 2007), p. xviii.

52. Norman Doidge, The Brain that Changes Itself (New York: The Penguin Group, 2007), p. 209.

LEARN MORE ABOUT ORIGINAL STRENGTH

Original Strength Systems (OS) is the leader in Nervous System Restoration and development of reflexive strength.

Our mission is to bring the hope and strength of movement to every body in the world. We provide accredited continuing education courses and books for health, fitness, and education professionals, empowering them to deliver better outcomes to their patients, clients, athletes, and students.

Based on the human developmental sequence, a series of movements that all humans naturally go through as they grow, and the human body's design, OS' Pressing RESET method teaches movements that help RESET an individual's neuromuscular system, allowing them to enjoy improved physical movement and physiological function.

If you want to learn more about Pressing RESET and reclaiming your original strength, https://originalstrength.net is your gateway. There, you'll discover a wealth of resources, from comprehensive books to hundreds of free video tutorials (OS Movement

Snax) and a complete directory of our courses and OS Certified Professionals in your vicinity.

We're here to support you every step of the way. If you're ready to enhance your movement system, we encourage you to connect with an OS Certified Professional. They can conduct an Original Strength Screen and Assessment (OSSA), a quick and straightforward method to identify areas for improvement. With the OSSA, the professional can guide you to the most effective starting point for your journey to restore your Original Strength through the Pressing RESET technique.

Remember, the OS team is always here for you. If you have any questions or need further guidance, please don't hesitate to reach out. We're committed to your journey towards better movement and health.

Please keep us updated on your progress. We want to know how you are doing. Progress@OriginalStrength.net

"…I am fearfully and wonderfully made…"
Psalm 139:14

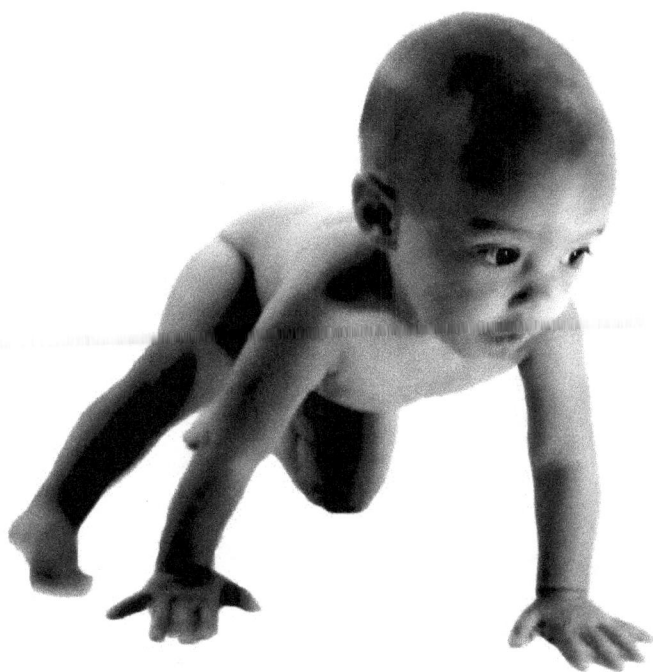